Essentials of Anatomy & Physiology Laboratory Manual

First Edition

David J. Hill

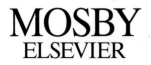

MOSBY
ELSEVIER

D0326160

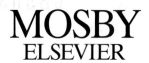

3251 Riverport Lane
St. Louis, Missouri 63043

ESSENTIALS OF ANATOMY & PHYSIOLOGY LAB MANUAL   ISBN: 978-0-323-05257-3

Notices

Knowledge and best practice in this field are constantly changing. As new research and experience broaden our understanding, changes in research methods, professional practices, or medical treatment may become necessary.

Practitioners and researchers must always rely on their own experience and knowledge in evaluating and using any information, methods, compounds, or experiments described herein. In using such information or methods they should be mindful of their own safety and the safety of others, including parties for whom they have a professional responsibility.

With respect to any drug or pharmaceutical products identified, readers are advised to check the most current information provided (i) on procedures featured or (ii) by the manufacturer of each product to be administered, to verify the recommended dose or formula, the method and duration of administration, and contraindications. It is the responsibility of practitioners, relying on their own experience and knowledge of their patients, to make diagnoses, to determine dosages and the best treatment for each individual patient, and to take all appropriate safety precautions.

To the fullest extent of the law, neither the Publisher nor the authors, contributors, or editors, assume any liability for any injury and/or damage to persons or property as a matter of products liability, negligence or otherwise, or from any use or operation of any methods, products, instructions, or ideas contained in the material herein.

Acquisitions Editor: Jeff Downing
Managing Editor: Becky Swisher
Sr. Developmental Editor: Karen Turner
Editorial Assistant: Chelsea Newton
Publishing Services Manager: Deborah Vogel
Design Manager: Teresa McBryan

Printed in the United States of America

Last digit is the print number: 9 8 7 6 5 4 3 2 1

Acknowledgments

I am very grateful for all of the support provided by the staff of Elsevier, including Jeff Downing, who was an enormous aide in materializing the ideas for this manual over the years; Rebecca Swisher, for steadfastly guiding the project to its completion; Karen Turner, for her patient efforts; Dan Matusiak, for filling the gaps; and Nadia Bidwell, who was invaluable in streamlining the manual and keeping my feet on the ground. Additionally, I would like to thank Blythe Nilson for her conversation and friendship beyond the call of duty.

Finally, I am grateful to be supported by my wife and best friend, Angel, who has offered encouragement, discussion and devotion throughout the process. Without her advice, this manual would not exist.

Preface

For many students, anatomy and physiology laboratory is their first hands-on experience learning about the human body. It is often a course of self-discovery as connections are made between anatomical structures and functions and the personal experience of being in your own skin. The course also involves engaging in scientific investigations in a laboratory environment. Many laboratory manuals have been written to guide students through this process, so what is different about this one?

The *Essentials in Anatomy & Physiology Laboratory Manual* makes a strong effort to connect scientific concepts to things students have experienced in their daily lives in our modern culture. In other words, this manual draws many analogies between the structures and functions of the human body and popular themes that are culturally accessible. This may involve teaching muscles and bones by having students think about superheroes or it may use military conflict to teach about the immune system.

This manual is not a textbook in the formal sense of the word. To streamline laboratory exercises and adapt to changes in laboratory environments, anatomy and physiology reference content is not included. This means that students *must* have access to a print textbook or online resource in order to access the relevant content during the labs. By opting to not repeat the same content in two places, it is hoped that the focus of the manual can be more streamlined to thematic exploration.

Ultimately, the goal of this manual is to provide a better bridge between anatomy and physiology concepts and what students already intuitively know about the body but may not actually realize that they know. Additionally, it is hoped that the analogies that are provided in this manual stimulate discussion so that anatomy and physiology can have broader applications and connections for students.

Manual Structure

Each unit begins with a relevant quote and conceptual introduction to the theme of the unit. Units and the exercise within them are organized according to principal body systems that should be familiar in the anatomy and physiology laboratory.

Sections in the manual are organized as exercises that contain laboratory activities. Each activity begins with an introduction, followed by relevant materials and safety issues.

A detailed procedure is provided for conducting each lab. The instructions may contain brief definitions, essential information about structures or functions, and necessary steps to complete the activity. The students will need to frequently access their textbooks to supplement the information provided in the procedures.

At the end of each exercise is the lab report where observations are recorded and sketches can be drawn. The lab report contains true/false, multiple-choice, and critical thinking questions relevant to the core material. While the true/false and multiple choice questions focus on recalling and understanding the content in the exercise, the critical thinking questions are geared toward connecting what was learned in the labs to the broader themes and analogies.

v

Your instructor may add to or modify any part of these exercises in order to best accommodate the laboratory environment, pedagogical requirements, or specific content he or she wants to cover. This may include dissections, which are not a part of the activities presented here, but are noted for the instructor in the Instructor's Manual.

Using This Manual

In order to complete laboratory exercises in this manual, you should:

1. Read the appropriate material in the textbook you are using for this course before you attend the laboratory.
2. Bring your textbook to the lab or ensure you have access to a comparable resource.
3. Prepare the materials for the lab activity you are assigned.
4. Ensure that you abide by safety rules as you follow the procedure.
5. Record your observations and data in the lab report.
6. Complete the lab report, answering any assigned questions.

Contents

Unit 1

Constituents of the Human Body

Holmes: *Then comes our expedition of today. By an examination of the ground I gained the trifling details… as to the personality of the criminal.*

Watson: *But how did you gain them?*

Holmes: *You know my method. It is founded upon the observation of trifles.*

—Sherlock Holmes in *The Boscombe Valley Mystery*

What is the appeal of crime drama?

Whether in books, radio, TV, or film, criminals and the law enforcement personnel that investigate their crimes are staples for storytellers. One of the first crime stories written, *The Tale of the Three Apples*, is part of a collection *One Thousand and One Nights* believed to contain tales dating from the 9th century. It tells of the mysterious death of a woman found in a chest, dismembered, and the investigation that discovers the real culprit among multiple men falsely confessing to the crime. Of all detectives, Sherlock Holmes is certainly one of the most famous and eccentric, using his keen observation and power of reason to unravel a mystery.

As you begin your study of anatomy and physiology, the human body may at times seem like a great mystery that requires you to push the limit of your rational abilities to understand. While you lean over a microscope examining tissue, you may find yourself relating to investigators on TV. You may find your investigation of cells and tissues to be driven by the same motives of detectives, either for a desire to know the truth or to appreciate the intricate details of a mastermind at work. Using crime drama as an analogy for the topics in Unit One can serve as a useful backdrop to help you better understand the limitless puzzles of the human body.

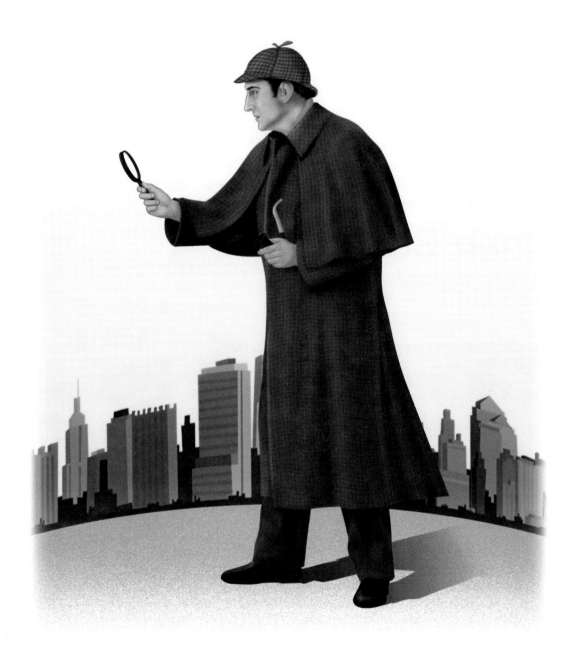

Exercise 1

Scientific Inquiry and the Human Body

Lesson Overview

Activity #1: Investigating the Proportionality Rule
Activity #2: The Scientific Method in Anatomy and Physiology
Activity #3: Error in Scientific Inquiry

Overview

For our first activity, we begin with an investigation into the proportionality of the human body to assess its general form before diving into the greater details of anatomy and physiology. This involves determining whether proportionality in the human body is universal. In the second activity you will conduct a scientific investigation into whether a mathematical ratio (the golden section) seen in nature is also found among various parts of the human body. Finally, you will assess the degree of error present in measurements of proportionality based on rules devised by Leonardo da Vinci.

Though the material in this exercise may not be covered in your textbook, understanding a bit about scientific inquiry will enhance your study of anatomy and physiology. Everything you need to know to correctly complete the labs for this exercise can be found in this unit.

Activity #1 — Investigating the Proportionality Rule

Introduction

Seeking to capture both the beauty and design of the human form, the 15th century artist Leonardo da Vinci was a detective in his own right, dabbling in the study of anatomy, including performing dissections on the dead. His investigations were fueled by a desire to understand both the aesthetics and mechanics of the human form. One of his most famous drawings, *Vitruvian Man*, was inspired by the first-century writings of Vitruvius, a Roman architect interested in proportionality. In his work, *De Architectura*, Vitruvius said the ideal human has the following proportions:

For if we measure the distance from the soles of the feet to the top of the head, and then apply that measure to the outstretched arms, the breadth will be found to be the same as the height, as in the case of plane surfaces which are perfectly square.

In other words, Vitruvius claimed that the human figure should fit exactly into a square, as the height and arm span length have a 1:1 ratio.

In this activity, you will measure the height and arm span length of fellow students in order to assess whether this proportionality rule is true.

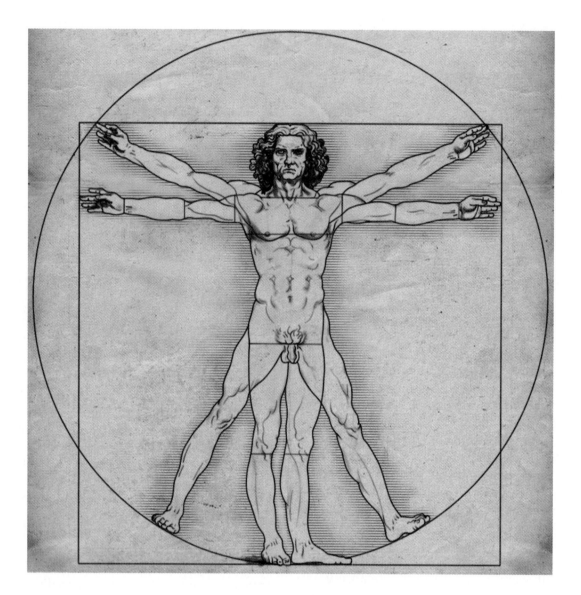

Materials

Tape measure
Calculator
Ruler

Before You Begin

- *All students will need to remove their shoes before being measured.*
- *All measurements should be made with a tape measure (a meter stick will not be long enough) and written in centimeters (cm).*
- *If the tape measure does not include the metric system, use the following conversions: 3.28 feet = 1 meter; 1 inch = 2.54 cm.*
- *You can calculate the ratio of any two body segments by measuring the length of each and dividing one measure into another. Whichever value you use as the denominator will be the "1" in your ratio. For example, if your arm span length is 164.0 cm and your height is 170.2 cm, your arm span-to-height ratio would be 0.96:1 (164.0/170.2).*
- *You will need to measure three to five male and three to five female subjects to accurately assess the proportionality rule.*

Procedure

1. For each subject, measure the height and arm span length with the tape measure and record your results. Calculate the ratio of arm span length to height.
2. Create a graph of your results using the total measured height (y-axis) and arm span length (x-axis). Use two different colored pens to differentiate between the male and female subject data.
3. A "best fit" line is an average that shows where points probably would be if there were no measurement errors. Use a ruler and draw two "best fit" lines — one for the male and one for the female data. Estimate the ratio of these lines.

Lab Report for 1.1

Section A. Activities for Investigating the Proportionality Rule

Subject name	Gender	Height (cm)	Arm span (cm)	Ratio

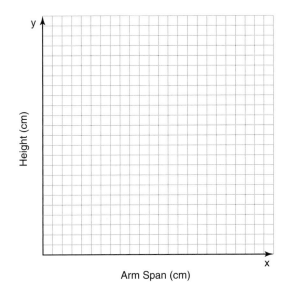

Arm Span (cm)

1. The proportionality rule of Vitruvius is 1:1 height to arm span length. Discuss the results you obtained from your investigation.

2. Was there a significant difference between male and female students? Should there be?

3. Vitruvius developed his rule on human proportionality 2,000 years ago. What do your results suggest about how the proportionality of the human body has changed in that time?

Section B. Assessments

1. T/F The forearm and foot have a 1:1 proportionality.
2. T/F The human figure can fit into a square but not a circle.
3. T/F According to Vitruvius, the human figure should fit exactly into a square because the height and arm span length have a 1:1 ratio.
4. An instructor informs a group of older students that they should notify her if anyone measures a proportionality ratio of more than 1.10 so that they can be tested for osteoporosis. One student who is 5'1" has an arm span length of 5'7". What can you conclude about these results?
    a. The student's proportionality ratio is over 1.10.
    b. The student's proportionality ratio is under 1.10.
    c. The student has osteoporosis.

Section C. Critical Thinking Problems

1. Vitruvius had a variety of other proportionality rules. For each of the following statements, describe how accurate you would expect it to be based on your own prior experience with the variability of the human body. Additionally, for each proportionality, express the fractional length provided as (i.) a ratio of the part being measured to the height and (ii.) a percent of the height.
    a. The head from the chin to the top is one-eighth of the height.

    b. The open hand from the wrist to the tip of the middle finger is a tenth of the height, while the forearm is one-fourth.

    c. The length of a foot is one-sixth the height.

2. Imagine that you are asked to take the stand as an expert in a criminal trial in which a man who is over seven feet tall is being prosecuted based solely on an impression in the mud of an enormous forearm. What argument would you make about the validity of the proportion of his forearm to his overall height?

Activity #2 — The Scientific Method in Anatomy and Physiology

Introduction

The scientific method is the process scientists use to conduct investigations and is best viewed as a set of reasoning guidelines. It is traditionally divided into five general stages: observation, hypothesis, experimentation, analysis, and conclusion.

Observation: Though often overlooked, the crucial first step in a scientific investigation is to observe something closely in an effort to understand what it is or how it works.

Hypothesis: A hypothesis is a preliminary answer to a question that emerges during the observation stage. It is an educated guess, but still speculation at this point.

Experimentation: Hypotheses are investigated through experimentation, which yields data, whether it is qualitative, such as descriptions, or quantitative, such as statistics.

Analysis: During analysis, data acquired through experimentation are evaluated for their relevance, validity, and repeatability. Patterns must be unearthed to find the essential data.

Conclusion: The conclusion to the scientific method is an assessment of whether the essential data that has been gathered supports the hypothesis or not. A hypothesis that has large amounts of data supporting it is well on its way to becoming a theory.

In order to get a better sense of how the scientific method applies to the study of the human body, you will propose and conduct your own investigation of a hypothesis related to one of the most fascinating patterns found in mathematics and in nature, the golden section or ratio (φ). Since the time of the ancient Greeks, this ratio has fascinated mathematicians and scientists as its value of approximately 1.61803 seems to recur throughout nature, even in quite unusual places, such as the shell of the nautilus or certain proportions of the human body.

Imagine that a scientist proposes that the golden section can be found throughout the proportions of the human body. The question is, "Which segments in the human body are proportional to the golden section?" To address this question, you will generate a hypothesis, conduct an investigation, and evaluate whether the data support the hypothesis.

Materials

Meter stick or tape measure
Calculator
Ruler

Before You Begin

- *Measurements less than a meter can be made with a meter stick; otherwise, use a tape measure.*
- *If the tape measure does not use the metric system, use the following conversions: 3.28 feet = 1 meter; 1 inch = 2.54 cm.*
- *You can calculate the ratio of any two body segments by measuring the length of each and dividing one measure into another. Whichever value you use as the denominator will be the "1" in your ratio.*

Procedure

1. Review the section in your textbook related to the scientific method.
2. For your preliminary observations, consider Figure 1.3, which shows geometric divisions of a human figure.
3. Determine which two measures have a ratio of approximately 1:1.6 and using this observation, generate a hypothesis in the following form:

In the human body, the proportion of the _____ to the _____ is the golden section.

4. Once you have your hypothesis, you will design an experiment to test it. Use your lab report to describe the plan for your investigation.

5. Clearly write out the steps of your procedure and the materials you will use.

6. Conduct the experiment and record the data in your lab report.

7. Analyze the data and determine whether it supports your hypothesis.

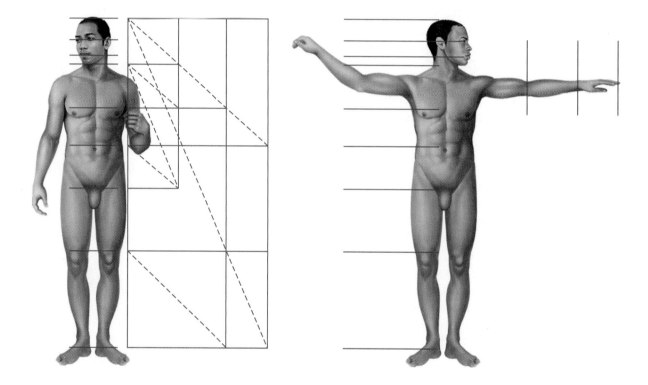

Figure 1.3 *Geometric divisions of the human body reflecting the ideal golden section. Measures include head to navel length : navel to foot length; knee to foot length : navel to knee length; eyes to mouth length : mouth to chin length; length of head : width of head; and length of hand : length of forearm.*

Lab Report for 1.2

Section A. Activities for the Scientific Method in Anatomy and Physiology

Describe the problem or ask a question

State the hypothesis

Design the experiment

Collect data

Conclusions

Hypothesis: *In the human body, the proportion of the _____ to the _____ is the golden section.*

Section B. Assessments

1. T/F Experimentation is necessary only when a hypothesis is known to be untrue.
2. T/F A hypothesis is written in the form of a question.
3. The analysis of data within the scientific method means to consider whether the data are:
   a. repeatable.
   b. relevant.
   c. valid.
   d. all of the above.
4. Match each term with the correct definition or explanation.
   a. theory
   b. experimentation
   c. hypothesis
   d. scientific method

   _____ A systematic approach to a scientific investigation

   _____ A hypothesis that is supported by a collection of reliable data

   _____ A process used to gather data to test a hypothesis

   _____ A reasonable answer to a question derived from previous observations

Section C. Critical Thinking Problems

1. From a scientific point of view, what benefit could come from understanding the proportionality of various parts of the human body?

2. Is a scientist who does not strictly follow the scientific method a fraud? Explain your answer.

Activity #3 — Error in Scientific Inquiry

Introduction

A trial offers an example of the scientific method. The prosecutor presents the hypothesis—the defendant is guilty. An argument is presented that includes observations and the results of inquiries, searches, interviews (all akin to experiments), which the prosecutor believes prove the hypothesis. It is up to the judge or jury to analyze the data in order to assess whether the hypothesis of guilt is supported, and come to a conclusion of guilt or innocence.

One study suggests that about 10,000 people per year are wrongly convicted of serious crimes. How does this happen? In a word: error. Errors like incorrect eyewitness reports, sloppy techniques used at the crime scene, poor arguments by either the prosecuting or defending attorneys or even simple bias on the part of the judge or jury.

Scientific investigations also contain errors that are classified as either random or systematic. Identifying, accounting for, and correcting errors are important parts of scientific inquiry, even though this step is not often formally recognized as part of the scientific method. It is especially important to assess error when a high degree of variability is present, such as with certain aspects of the human body.

In this activity, you will assess the error in the proportions that da Vinci used when he drew *Vitruvian Man*.

Materials

Tape measure
Ruler
Calculator

Procedure

1. In describing the proportionality of the ideal human body, da Vinci came up with the following generalized rules:
   - Four fingers (width) make one palm
   - Six palms (width) make one cubit (defined as the forearm length)
   - Four cubits make a man's height
   Therefore, each person's height should be equivalent to 96 finger-widths or 24 palm-widths.
2. Record your actual height in centimeters in your lab report. Have a partner use a tape measure to measure your height if you do not know it.
3. Measure the width of each finger and your palm using a ruler and record your results in your lab report.
4. Calculate your height based on each measurement by multiplying the width of each finger by 96 and the width of your palm by 24.
5. Compare this height to your actual height.
6. You can calculate the percentage of error in your measurements using the following formula:

$$\frac{\text{calculated height} - \text{actual height}}{\text{actual height}} \times 100\% = \underline{\quad}\% \text{ error}$$

Lab Report for 1.3

Section A. Activities for Error in Scientific Inquiry

Actual height: _____ (cm)

	Width (cm)		Calculated height (cm)	Percent error
Index finger		x 96 =		
Middle finger		x 96 =		
Ring finger		x 96 =		
Little finger		x 96 =		
Palm		x 24 =		

1. Name one source of error in this experiment.

2. How does the variability in the width of your fingers affect your calculated heights?

3. How much variability is there between your finger and palm widths and a partner's? Explain how this might affect your results.

4. Are da Vinci's rules accurate?

Section B. Assessments

1. T/F A cubit is a precise measure of length.
2. T/F Errors in experimental data can be classified as either random or systematic.
3. If the length of an individual's foot is the same as the forearm length, how many finger-widths long is a foot?
   a. 4
   b. 16
   c. 24
   d. 96

Section C. Critical Thinking Problems

1. What are some of the problems with profiling perpetrators based on estimated height, weight and stature?

2. Respond to the following statement: *While error is important to consider in the sciences, anatomy is error-free because it is an exact science.*

3. Should experimental results that contain errors always be excluded during analysis? Think about the nature of error and how error is detected in your response.

Exercise 2

Organization of the Body and the Language of Anatomy

Overview

Rarely do movies or TV shows depict detectives as being short on skills at the scene of a crime. They'll check a man who is on the ground bleeding and say, "He's been shot in the shoulder, but he'll be all right." The level of expertise demonstrated in this rapid-fire medical assessment may seem natural for a TV detective, but in the real world, the ability to properly communicate about the human body is not a skill one easily picks up "on the beat."

Anatomical terminology is highly sophisticated, with a long tradition rooted in the Greek and Latin languages. It not only defines regions and specific locations, but directions, positions, and orientations, allowing for anyone, regardless of where they live or the language they speak, to navigate around the entire body with precision. Anatomical terminology is usually associated with medical professionals but everyone can benefit from knowing basic terms, even if they aren't on *CSI*.

To begin your study of anatomical terms, we will review the levels of organization in the body and common organ systems. Then we will define terms related to common reference points on the exterior of the body and proceed within it, while introducing terminology related to navigating through the body.

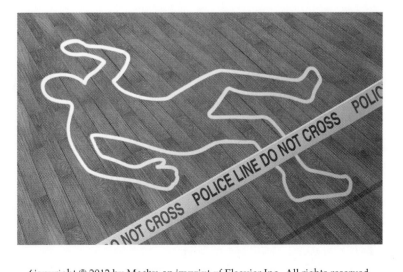

17

Activity #1 — Levels of Organization and Organ Systems

Materials

Model of the human body with organ systems
Posters of the levels of organization and organ systems

Introduction

A criminal investigation is often a complex exercise in problem solving. Investigators may start off knowing little about a crime other than the fact that it occurred. As they gather evidence, a picture of the crime emerges. Details as minute as a strand of hair or an odd stain can be as significant to the crime's eventual solution as a statement from a witness.

Understanding how the human body works bears similarities to a criminal investigation. Events that occur at the molecular level can be as important as those happening to an organ system. Unraveling all of these connections requires a general sense of the "crime scene," that is, the human body and all that it contains.

To accomplish this, we begin by examining the levels of organization in the body from the molecular level to organ systems. After having a general review of the organ systems, we'll be ready to collect more evidence in the activities that follow.

Procedure

1. Review the section in your textbook related to levels of organization and organ systems in the human body.
2. To understand many of the structures and processes occurring in the body, you will need to be able to change the scale under consideration rapidly. Identify the levels of organization by correctly labeling the structures in Figure 2.2.
3. To gain a general sense of the location and distribution of organ systems in the body, identify the organs systems shown in Figure 2.2.

Lab Report for 2.1

Section A. Activities for Levels of Organization and Organ Systems

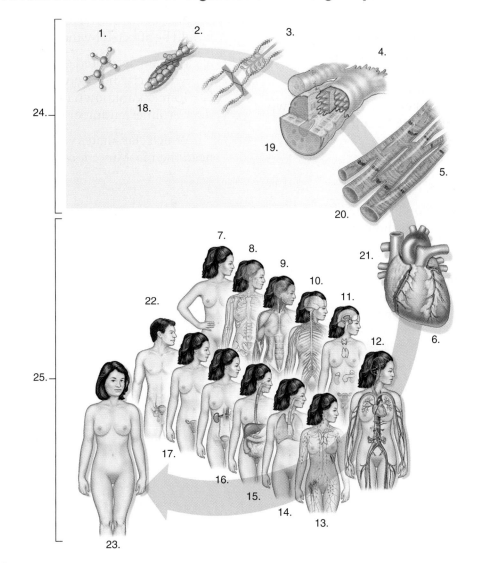

Figure 2.2

Relevant Terms		
_____ Atom	_____ Integumentary	_____ Organism level
_____ Cardiovascular	_____ Lymphatic	_____ Protein filaments
_____ Cellular level	_____ Microscopic level	_____ Reproductive
_____ Chemical level	_____ Molecule	_____ Respiratory
_____ Digestive	_____ Muscular	_____ Skeletal
_____ Endocrine	_____ Nervous	_____ The heart
_____ Gross level	_____ Organ level	_____ Tissue level
_____ Heart muscle cell	_____ Organ system level	_____ Urinary
_____ Heart muscle tissue		

Section B. Assessments

1. T/F The cell is the smallest structural unit of the body that is alive.
2. The level of organization in the body from smallest to largest is:
   a. cellular, molecular, tissue, organ.
   b. molecular, cellular, tissue, organ.
   c. molecular, tissue, cellular, organ.
   d. molecular, cellular, organ, tissue.
3. The term most likely derived from two Greek words meaning "a cutting up" is:
   a. physiology.
   b. homeostasis.
   c. anatomy.
   d. organization.
4. Which of the following organ systems is NOT distributed throughout the entire body?
   a. Digestive system
   b. Lymphatic system
   c. Integumentary system
   d. Cardiovascular system

Section C. Critical Thinking Problem

1. Imagine a severe earthquake strikes and a number of your classmates have been injured.

   Name all of the organ systems that would be affected by the following injuries:

   a. William: lacerated ear
   b. Sylvia: crushed pelvic region
   c. Tom: an unknown neck injury
   d. Caroline: a number of broken toes

   Which classmates would you speculate need the most urgent care?

Activity #2 — Major Regions, Landmarks, and Cavities

Materials

Human torso models
Posters of the major regions, landmarks and cavities
Colored pencils or markers

Introduction

Before the invention of noninvasive technologies that allow doctors and scientists to peer inside the body, information about anatomy was obtained through dissections. The Egyptian Herophilus (335-280 B.C.) is credited as the first to systematically dissect human cadavers as well as animals. Dubbed the "Father of Anatomy," he wrote extensively about his work (in books which are now lost) and later founded the great medical school in Alexandria.

After Herophilus, human dissection was banned by the Roman Empire and would remain so for 1,800 years. It would be the Flemish physician Andreas Vesalius in the 16th century who would take up the practice of dissection again and wrote the first anatomy textbooks. As the modern Father of Anatomy, Vesalius conducted his work for the sake of education while artists around the same time, such as Leonardo da Vinci and Michelangelo, dissected cadavers to gain knowledge of the human form for their artistic depictions. For 500 years, education in the anatomical sciences has been deeply rooted in human dissection.

Fortunately, the body can be divided into general regions, such as the cranial or abdominal regions, which facilitates focus on the specific area being considered. Furthermore, the exterior of the body has surface landmarks that are easy to identify and help when referencing internal structures. Many of the organ systems are compartmentalized within certain cavities of the body, which can help you understand their interrelationships.

As sophisticated as medical terminology has become, common reference points are a vital part of the language of anatomy. In this activity, you will identify some of the important regions, landmarks, and cavities of the body used in anatomical vernacular.

Before You Begin

- *As you work to identify features in the diagrams, be sure to identify them on your own body and/or on a partner's when possible. This will provide you with another way to remember these anatomical terms.*

Procedure

1. Review the section in your textbook related to regions, landmarks, and cavities of the body.
2. Features of the body that serve as reference points are important when discussing anatomy. Some of these terms may be familiar. Identify the common landmarks and regions of the body indicated in Figure 2.3 using the terms provided.
3. Certain organ systems are segregated from others within compartments called *cavities*. Label the cavities in Figure 2.4 using the terms provided.

Lab Report for 2.2

Section A. Activities for Major Regions, Landmarks, and Cavities

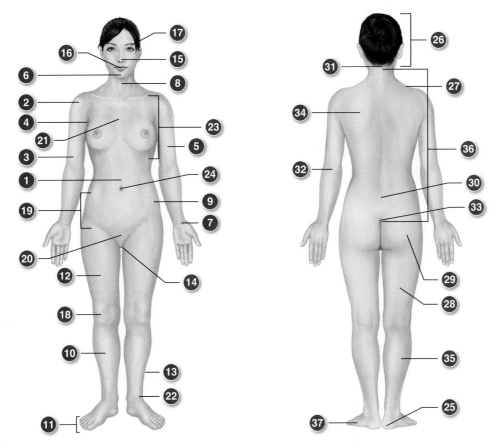

Figure 2.3

Relevant Terms		
Anterior Body Landmarks		**Posterior Body Landmarks**
_____ Abdominal	_____ Fibular	_____ Calcaneal
_____ Acromial	_____ Inguinal	_____ Cephalic
_____ Antecubital	_____ Nasal	_____ Deltoid
_____ Axillary	_____ Oral	_____ Femoral
_____ Brachial	_____ Orbital	_____ Gluteal
_____ Buccal	_____ Patellar	_____ Lumbar
_____ Carpal	_____ Pelvic	_____ Occipital
_____ Cervical	_____ Pubic	_____ Olecranal
_____ Coxal	_____ Sternal	_____ Plantar
_____ Crural	_____ Tarsal	_____ Popliteal
_____ Digital	_____ Thoracic	_____ Scapular
_____ Femoral	_____ Umbilical	_____ Sural
		_____ Vertebral

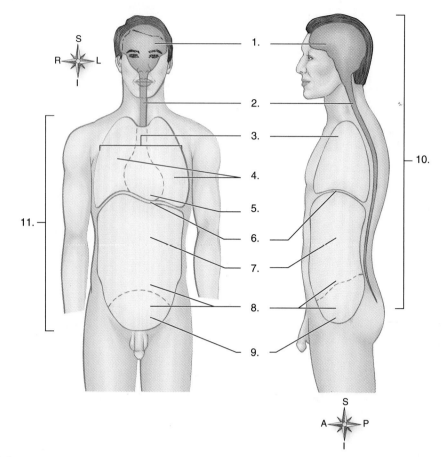

Figure 2.4

Relevant Terms	
_____ Abdominal cavity	_____ Pelvic cavity
_____ Abdominopelvic cavity	_____ Pleural cavities
_____ Cranial cavity	_____ Spinal cavity
_____ Diaphragm	_____ Thoracic cavity
_____ Dorsal body cavity	_____ Ventral body cavity
_____ Mediastinum	

1. In the following figure, color in the different regions of the body and write their corresponding names from the list provided.

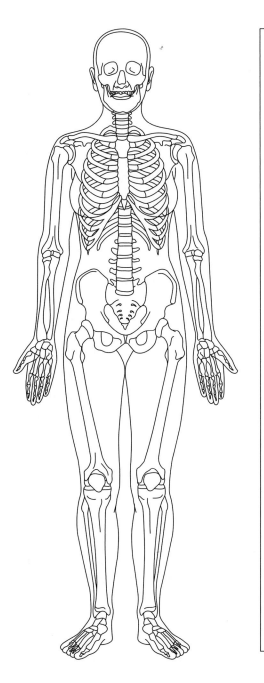

Cephalic
Cervical
Thoracic
Brachial
Antebrachial
Carpal
Manual
Abdominal
Lumbar
Gluteal
Pelvic
Pubic
Inguinal
Femoral
Crural
Sural
Tarsal
Pedal
Plantar

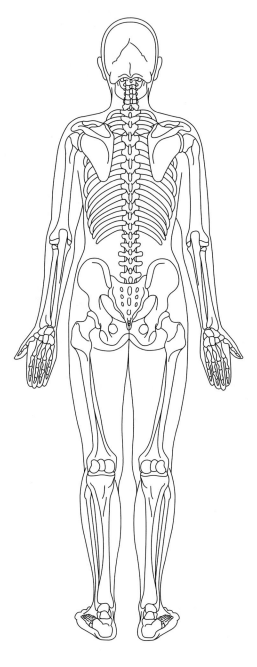

2. You come upon a crime scene where a victim has been severely beaten. State the regions, landmarks or body cavities in which wounds are located. Use the following illustration to guide you:

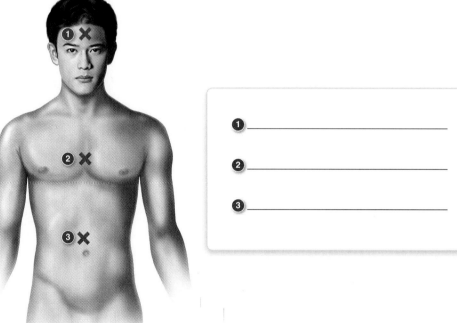

1 _____

2 _____

3 _____

Figure 2.6

Section B. Assessments

1. T/F The antebrachial, umbilical, and left lumbar regions are all in the middle abdominopelvic area.
2. T/F The term "leg" only refers to the portion of the lower limb between the knee and the ankle.
3. The diaphragm separates the:
   a. dorsal from the ventral cavity.
   b. abdominal from the pelvic cavity.
   c. thoracic from the abdominal cavity.
   d. pleural from the mediastinum.
4. Which of the following does NOT describe a part of the head region?
   a. olecranal
   b. temporal
   c. zygomatic
   d. buccal
5. Which of the following structures acts as a physical barrier between the pelvic cavity and the abdominal cavity?
   a. mediastinum
   b. mesenteries
   c. diaphragm
   d. none of the above

6. The olecranal is to upper extremity as the _____ is to the lower extremity.
   a. popliteal
   b. gluteal
   c. inguinal
   d. plantar

Section C. Critical Thinking Problems

1. Which of the body features in Figure 2.6 are at fixed locations? General regions?

2. What are the advantages and disadvantages of segregated cavities?

Activity #3 — System of Terminology and Anatomical Relationships

Introduction

We reference anatomy in our day-to-day speech, such as when we say someone is a *pain in the neck*. But colloquialisms lack the specificity required in a scientific system referring to the body and all it contains. For anatomical terminology to be effective and accurate, it must accomplish three things.

First, we want to be able to consistently find a particular feature on any given person. It doesn't do a sketch artist any good for a witness to say that a suspect had a scar "somewhere" on his face; referencing regions and landmarks helps to identify particular aspects of a person's body.

Second, we need a singular reference position for the body, so that when we talk about an organ, the liver for instance, we can easily talk about where it is relatively located, whether in another person or our own body. The reference position commonly used is the anatomical position, which involves a person standing upright facing the observer with the hands at the sides and palms facing outward.

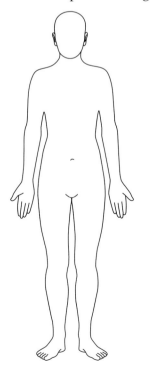

Third, we want to be able to describe the spatial relationships between anatomical features. While the phrase "leg bone connected to the knee bone" might be acceptable for a children's song, it is obviously inadequate for the precision needed in anatomy. We need to be able to describe the relative position or orientation of one anatomical feature *to* another precisely, such as the heart is *medial to* the lungs.

To accomplish these three things, anatomical language consists of the following:

- Terminology for components that follow consistent sets of naming rules that indicate location or function
- Terminology for relative position, direction and orientation
- Terminology for spatial relationships related to planes and sections

In this activity, we will delve into the language of anatomy and begin building the vocabulary needed to speak accurately about the human body.

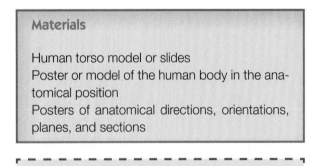

Materials

Human torso model or slides
Poster or model of the human body in the anatomical position
Posters of anatomical directions, orientations, planes, and sections

Before You Begin

- *As you learn this system of terminology, keep in mind that the language of anatomy was developed for the purpose of communication. For this reason, it is important to practice using this language, as you would with any language, to ensure that you know what the terms are describing and that you are using them in the proper context.*

Procedure

1. Review the section in your textbook related to anatomical orientations, directions, planes, and sections.

2. Describing the orientation of one feature to another can be accomplished with directional terminology. In some cases, it's also necessary use directional terms that reference certain natural planes in the body, such as the sagittal plane afforded by bilateral symmetry. Match the terms in Figure 2.8 with the correct directions and planes in the body.

3. Two systems of reference are used to divide the abdominopelvic cavity into either four quadrants or nine regions. Identify both sets of abdominopelvic subdivisions in Figure 2.9.

Section A. Activities for System of Terminology and Anatomical Relationships

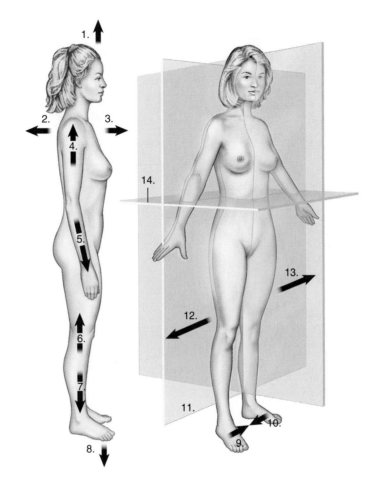

Figure 2.8

Relevant Terms	
_____ Anterior	_____ Medial
_____ Distal	_____ Posterior
_____ Distal	_____ Proximal
_____ Frontal plane	_____ Proximal
_____ Inferior	_____ Sagittal plane
_____ Lateral	_____ Superior
_____ Lateral	_____ Transverse plane
_____ Medial	

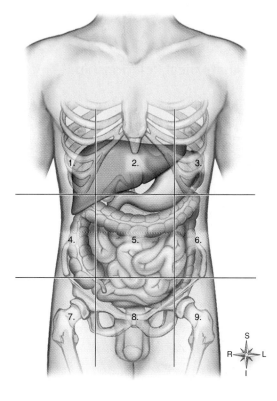

Relevant Terms
_____ Epigastric region
_____ Hypogastric region
_____ Left hypochondriac region
_____ Left Iliac (inguinal) region
_____ Left lumbar region
_____ Right hypochondriac region
_____ Right Iliac (inguinal) region
_____ Right lumbar region
_____ Umbilical region

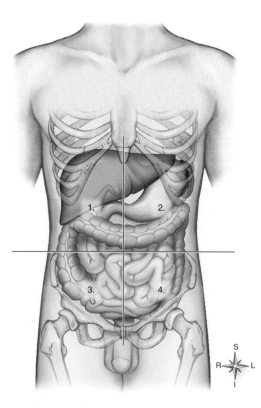

Relevant Terms
_____ Left lower
_____ Left upper
_____ Right lower
_____ Right upper

Figure 2.9

1. Use the numbers in the following illustration to identify the directional terms listed in the Relevant Terms box.

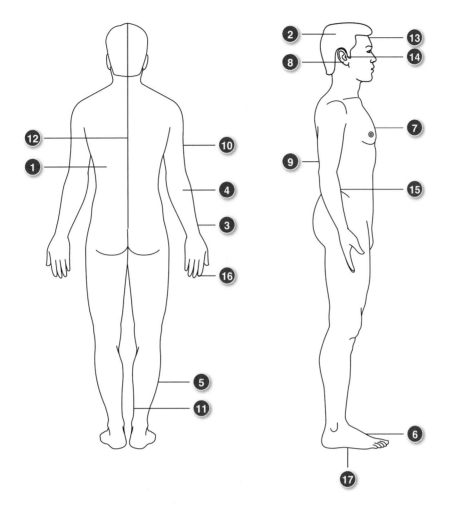

Relevant Terms	
_____ Anterior surface of arm	_____ Lateral surface of leg
_____ Anterior surface of head	_____ Medial surface of arm
_____ Distal portion of hand	_____ Medial surface of leg
_____ Dorsal surface of trunk	_____ Posterior surface of arm
_____ Inferior surface of ear	_____ Proximal portion of hand
_____ Inferior surface of foot	_____ Superior portion of ear
_____ Lateral surface of arm	_____ Ventral surface of trunk
_____ Lateral surface of head	

2. With the advent of radiologic techniques like CAT scans and MRI, we are able to see through the body in sections. However, some of these images can be disorienting. To help understand how an object appears from different planes and sections, identify where the slices of banana shown came from on the whole banana. In Figure 2.11, draw a line from each slice of banana to the plane from which it was cut.

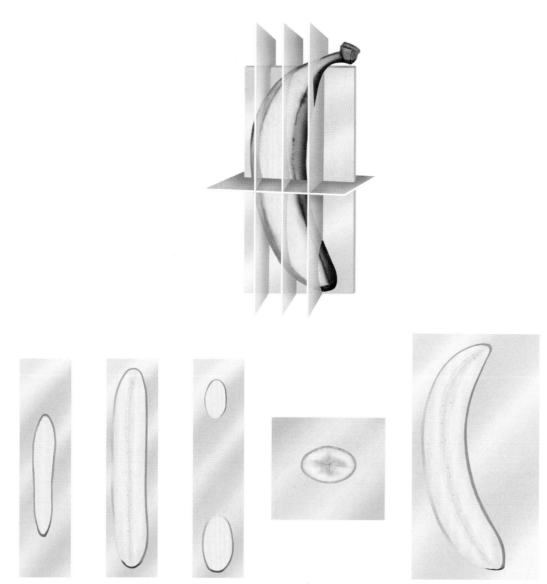

Figure 2.11

3. You are reading through a surgeon's report on a patient. In the report, the surgeon indicated that she made the following incisions:

- Incision 1: Made in the left anterior thoracic cavity, five centimeters lateral to the trachea and three centimeters superior to the diaphragm; the incision extended eight centimeters inferior to the abdominal region.
- Incision 2: Located in the right anterior axillary region, extending medially to the mediastinum. At the mediastinum, the incision turned inferiorly to six centimeters superior to the right iliac region.
- Incision 3: At the right posterior scapular region, the incision extended medially to four centimeters lateral to the vertebral region, where it turned inferiorly two centimeters to the lumbar region.

Use the following outlines of the human body to draw these incisions as described.

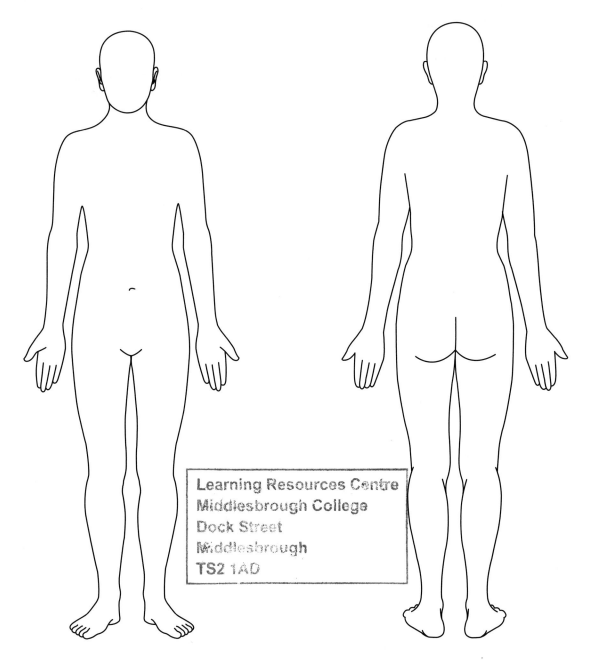

Section B. Assessments

1. T/F   The antonym of medial is proximal.
2. T/F   All body directional terms use the supine position when referencing positions.
3. T/F   The ankle is distal to the knee.
4. A slice that divides the body into anterior and posterior portions is called the:
    a. transverse plane.
    b. sagittal plane.
    c. frontal plane.
    d. none of the above.
5. A doctor is describing an MRI scan made through the center of the head with both the right and left eyes in the scan. The plane that was scanned is the:
    a. coronal plane.
    b. midsagittal plane.
    c. transverse plane.
    d. both a and c.
6. In the human body, _____ means the same as ventral.
    a. anterior
    b. superior
    c. medial
    d. proximal

Section C. Critical Thinking Problems

1. If the language of anatomy is so accurate, why isn't it a standard part of English? What are the pros and cons of using accurate language in everyday speech?

2. You are an emergency medical technician. Explain why it would be important for you to use the language of anatomy when describing a patient's injuries.

Exercise 3

Inner World of the Cell

Lesson Overview

Activity #1: Cell Structure and Function
Activity #2: DNA Extraction and Analysis
Activity #3: Transport in the Cell
  Part A: Brownian Motion
  Part B: Diffusion
  Part C: Osmosis
Activity #4: Life Cycle of the Cell

Overview

On a day-to-day basis, we rarely have reason to think about what the cells within our bodies are up to, yet science has devoted vast quantities of time to investigating cells and new breakthroughs in understanding them continue. Advances in science and medicine continue to show that what happens at the cellular level has enormous impact on the organismal level. But this was not always understood. In the late 17th century when Robert Hooke and Anton van Leeuwenhoek used primitive microscopes to look at cellular life for the first time, they began a branch of science that has become increasingly important over the last 300 years. Though scientists have ventured deeply into its inner workings, the cell continues to hold a host of mysteries that demand investigation.

To begin the study of the cell, we start by examining the common structures within a typical cell and their functions in an effort to unravel their role in specific cellular processes. Then we will investigate cellular physiology, specifically in the area of transport. Finally, we will examine the development of the cell throughout its life cycle.

Activity #1 — Cell Structure and Function

Introduction

After the isolated homicide or serial killer case, any good Hollywood detective ultimately confronts organized crime. The detective must collect evidence about an organization, putting the pieces together to determine the scope and scale of its illegal activity. A detective might have to go undercover to learn everything about the organization from the inside. Members must be identified, their purposes and ranks within the hierarchy understood, and all illegal activities cataloged in an effort to take down the leader.

In a sense, the cell can be thought of as a criminal organization. It is a complex system of molecular species arranged within a hierarchy to accomplish several key functions vital for its survival, namely:

1. A cell must be able to acquire the resources it needs to carry out processes and build necessary components.
2. A cell must be able to monitor, correct and/or adapt to any threatening situations that could jeopardize its well-being.
3. A cell must be able to develop independently and generate new cells without necessarily destroying the original cell.

Like a detective attempting to resolve the inner workings of organized crime, your task is to decipher the activity within the cell by identifying structures, describing their roles in processes, and connecting all the activities back to the cell's primary functions.

Materials

Eukaryotic cell models
Microscope
Slides of eukaryotic cellular components

Procedure

1. Review the content in your textbook related to the cell and cellular components.
2. The cell consists of:
   a. a plasma membrane, which is a double layer of phospholipids containing cholesterol and embedded proteins that serves as the cellular barrier to the external environment
   b. organelles, a variety of smaller structures that serve specialized functions within eukaryotic cells
   c. cytoplasm, the jelly-like matrix that supports the organelles

   Using the terms provided, label the cellular structures in Figure 3.1.
3. Examine slides of eukaryotic cells with a microscope. Sketch what you observe in the areas provided in the lab report and label as many organelles as you can.
4. Match the structures of the cell with the functions and descriptions listed in the appropriate section of your lab report.
5. Human flora is the total collection of microorganisms that exist in and around the tissues of the human body, located especially in the gastrointestinal tract. Many of these microorganisms are simpler prokaryotes like bacteria though some are eukaryotes like fungi, especially yeast. As you study cellular components, keep in mind that within your body lie both species of eukaryotic cells.

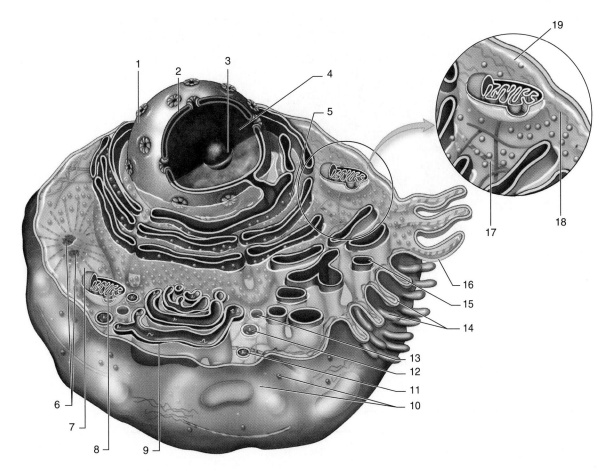

Figure 3.1

Relevant Terms		
_____ Centrioles	_____ Lysosome	_____ Nucleolus
_____ Centrosome	_____ Microfilament	_____ Nucleus
_____ Chromatin	_____ Microtubule	_____ Peroxisome
_____ Cilia	_____ Microvilli	_____ Rough endoplasmic reticulum
_____ Cytoskeleton	_____ Mitochondrion	_____ Smooth endoplasmic reticulum
_____ Free ribosomes	_____ Nuclear envelope	_____ Vesicle
_____ Golgi apparatus		

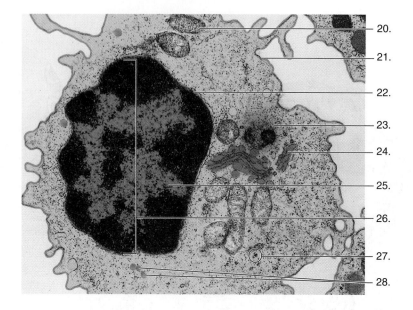

20.

21.

22.

23.

24.

25.

26.

27.

28.

Figure 3.1

Relevant Terms	
_____ Centrosome	_____ Nuclear membrane
_____ Chromatin	_____ Nucleus
_____ Golgi apparatus	_____ Plasma membrane
_____ Mitochondrion	_____ Ribosomes

Lab Report for 3.1

Section A. Activities for Cell Structure and Function

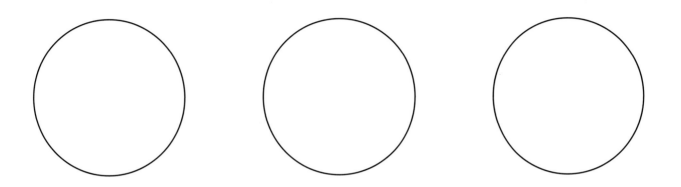

1. Match each cell structure with its correct description or function.

_____ centriole	a. exterior boundary of the cell consisting of phospholipids, cholesterol, and proteins
_____ cilia	b. cellular fluid between the plasma membrane and the nucleus that supports organelles
_____ cytoplasm	c. granules that are the site of protein synthesis
_____ endoplasmic reticulum	d. elongated organelles that contain their own DNA and produce the energy required by the cell to function
_____ flagella	e. a system of interconnected membranes important in transport that may be embedded with ribosomes (making them 'rough' as opposed to 'smooth')
_____ Golgi apparatus	f. stacks of smooth membrane sacs involved in protein packaging for transport
_____ lysosome	g. sac-like organelles containing enzymes for chemical digestion
_____ mitochondria	h. tubular structures that play an important role in cell division
_____ nucleolus	i. short hair-like structures that help move substances across the surface of some cells
_____ nucleus	j. long, tail-like extension that is the primary means of motion in sperm cells
_____ plasma membrane	k. organelle that contains cellular DNA and plays a role in controlling numerous cellular functions including cell transport, metabolism, and growth
_____ ribosome	l. part of the nucleus that aids in the formation of ribosomes

2. For each of the cellular processes listed below, create a flow chart of the structures involved, describe their role and use arrows to show the "flow" of the process.
   a. Translation and transcription
   b. Exocytosis
   c. Cellular respiration

Section B. Assessments

1. T/F   Ribosomes are the "power plants" of the cells.
2. T/F   Embedded ribosomes make rough endoplasmic reticulum rough.
3. The plasma membrane of a cell consists of:
   a. proteins.
   b. phospholipids.
   c. cholesterol molecules.
   d. all of the above.
4. The organelle in the cell that controls most of the activities is the:
   a. cilia.
   b. nucleus.
   c. nucleolus.
   d. ribosomes.
5. Which organelle in the cell contains its own DNA?
   a. mitochondrion
   b. endoplasmic reticulum
   c. Golgi apparatus
   d. centriole

Section C. Critical Thinking Problem

1. Prokaryotes lack the compartmentalization that organelles afford to eukaryotes, yet these cells are still able to thrive and accomplish many of the same functions that eukaryotic cells can, such as metabolism, reproduction, and growth. What is the advantage then of segregating certain components in eukaryotic cells into organelles?

Activity #2 — DNA Extraction and Analysis

Introduction

Much like the head of a criminal organization, nuclear DNA can be thought of as the crime boss in the eukaryotic cellular world. After all, it has its own special enclosure within the cell to protect it from harm and other cellular components. It communicates with the rest of the cell only through messengers, mRNA, and these orders dictate what the cell must produce. Finally, it hordes the best "loot" in the form of genetic information needed to produce the proteins vital to the cell.

When we think of our own DNA in our cells, it may seem like an elusive molecule—something that we know is there, but that we can never get our hands on. But just as relentless investigators know, capturing the crime boss is deeply satisfying. In this experiment, you will isolate some of your own DNA, getting your hands on it once and for all.

Materials

Paper cup
Sterilized cotton swabs (as an alternative to mouth rinsing)
Test tubes
Glass rod
Meat tenderizer
Filter paper
Hot plates
Chromatography vessel
UV Lamp or cabinet
0.9% NaCl solution or light-colored Gatorade
25% liquid detergent solution
Chilled ethanol (95% or 190 proof) or isopropyl alcohol
1 M HCl
1:4:2 acetic acid:isopropyl alcohol:water, by volume

Before You Begin

- *Your instructor may choose to have you acquire cheek cells using a sterilized cotton swab rather than through mouth rinsing. If that is the case, you can acquire the cells by dabbing the sterilized cotton swab on the inside of your cheeks a few times then swirl the tip of the swab in the solution in step 1.*
- *Your instructor may choose to have you acquire DNA from your hair follicles as a way of investigating forensic techniques. It may be necessary, however, to use a microscope to see the DNA. Hair itself does not contain DNA but the hair follicles do. Acquire approximately a dozen of your hairs with the follicles attached and separate the shafts from the follicles. Add these follicles to the test tube described in step d of the DNA acquisition procedure and proceed.*

Procedure

1. Review the content in your textbook related to the structure of DNA.
2. Use the following procedure for **DNA acquisition:**
   a. Pour 10 mL (2 teaspoons) of either a 0.9% NaCl solution or light-colored Gatorade into a paper cup.
   b. Vigorously swirl the liquid in your mouth for 30 seconds in order to remove cheek cells. It will help to gently rub your teeth against your cheeks to help remove more cells (the more cells, the more DNA).
   c. Spit the solution into the paper cup.
   d. Pour this solution into a test tube containing 1 mL (1/4 teaspoon) of a 25% liquid detergent solution.
   e. Rock the test tube gently back and forth for about 3 minutes, which will cause the cells to rupture. Do not shake too vigorously as it breaks apart the DNA strands and will minimize the amount of extract.

f. Dissolve a very small amount (less than a pinch) of meat tenderizer into the test tube. The meat tenderizer contains enzymes that break down proteins attached to DNA.

g. Allow the solution to sit for 5 minutes.

3. Use the following procedure for **DNA separation**:

a. Carefully pour 5 mL of chilled ethanol (95% or 190 proof) or isopropyl alcohol along the inside of the tube. It will form a layer on top of the soap solution.

b. Allow the tube to sit undisturbed for 1 minute.

c. Insert a glass rod, elongated paper clip, or narrow tweezers into the tube such that the tip penetrates the boundary layer between the ethanol and the soap solution.

d. Begin to turn the rod or paper clip in one direction, which will cause DNA strands to wind around the tip. If the DNA was physically damaged, it will form clumps around the tip.

e. Place the spooled DNA into another test tube containing 5 mL of ethanol for storage.

4. While you may have obtained material from the separation procedure above, some instructors may opt for you to prove that it is DNA. To do so, use the following procedure for **DNA degradation and analysis** (alternatively, this may be done as a class demonstration by your instructor):

a. Decant the 5 mL of ethanol from the test tube.

b. Add 5 mL of water to the test tube and swirl until the DNA dissolves.

c. Add 1.0 mL of 1 M HCl to the test tube and heat it for 10 minutes in boiling water.

d. Remove the tube from the water and allow it too cool.

e. Using the tip of a glass pipette, place a small drop of the solution onto a strip of filter paper suitable for paper chromatography. Allow the spots to dry before proceeding.

f. Insert the paper into a chromatography vessel which contains a small amount of solvent (a solution of 1:4:2 acetic acid:isopropyl alcohol:water, by volume), making sure that the DNA spot is not below the solvent line. Cap the vessel.

g. Using a UV lamp or cabinet, monitor the migration of the spots up the paper. The approximate time required to do this will vary. The spots correspond to the four nucleotides in DNA and should follow the order, from longest migration to shortest, of guanine, adenine, cytosine, and thymine.

Lab Report for 3.2

Section A. Activities for DNA Extraction and Analysis

1. Describe your observations during the DNA separation stage of the experiment.

2. Describe your observations during the DNA degradation and analysis stage of the experiment.

Section B. Assessments

1. T/F   The basic building block of DNA is nucleotides.
2. The "deoxy" part of deoxyribonucleic acid refers to which component of its structure?
   a. nucleotides
   b. phosphate groups
   c. sugar backbone
3. A student tries to isolate DNA from his hair. After conducting the acquisition and separation steps, no DNA was observed by the student. Which of the following could explain why this occurred?
   a. It can only be visualized with a UV lamp.
   b. The hair used was a clipping from a recent haircut.
   c. This student does not have any DNA.

Section C. Critical Thinking Problems

1. Based on the experiment you conducted, is DNA well-protected or vulnerable inside of eukaryotic cells?

2. To a degree, it can be disappointing to obtain your DNA and find that it looks like white string. Many of the illustrations and animations we see of DNA show this amazing three-dimensional architecture. In the end, what is a more effective way of helping everyone understand DNA: visually depicting it and/or actually obtaining it yourself?

Activity #3 — Transport in the Cell

Part A: Brownian Motion

Introduction

Understanding transport and exchange processes of molecules is a vital part to unraveling how the cell functions. The simplest type of motion in the cell occurs even in the smallest molecules. Their motion is chaotic and patternless and is known as *Brownian motion* after the botanist Robert Brown who described the random movement of pollen particles in water in 1827:

> "While examining the form of these [particles of pollen grains] immersed in water, I observed many of them very evidently in motion; their motion consisting not only of a change in place in the fluid manifested by alterations in their relative positions... *These motions were such as to satisfy me, after frequently repeated observations, that they arose neither from currents in the fluid, nor from its gradual evaporation [convection], but belonged to the particle itself.*"
>
> —Robert Brown, *Microscopic Observations on the Pollen of Plants*

In 1905, Albert Einstein determined that the motion that Brown described occurred in the molecules of the liquid, in which the different kinetic energies of the molecules and their varying orientations caused them to move in random directions and collide chaotically. Organelles and other cellular components that are not anchored down demonstrate Brownian motion such as moving randomly in a circle or from one side of the cell to the other.

Because this motion is present and is a natural transport process within the cell, it is worth investigating in its own right.

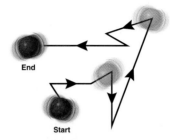

End

Start

Materials

Metal tray
Glass marbles (many small marbles and a few large marbles)
Wet mount slide
Distilled water
Medicine droppers
India ink
Whole milk
Microscope with 200x or 400x magnification
Slides cover slips

Procedure

1. Review the content in your textbook related to Brownian motion.
2. A simple way to model Brownian motion is to place a large amount of small marbles and a few larger marbles in a metal tray. Move the tray side-to-side or forward-and-backward within a two-dimensional plane in order to create random motion of marbles. As you do so, observe the motion of the larger marbles relative to the smaller ones.
3. To observe Brownian motion with a chemical substance, place a droplet of India ink, which is a colloidal suspension of carbon particles in various solvents, onto a slide, place a drop of water onto the ink and cover with a cover slip.
4. Using the microscope, examine the ink droplets. Allow the suspension to sit for a few minutes until all the motion becomes random.
5. Using the spaces provided in your lab report, select one globule and trace its motion over a 30-second period.
6. Repeat the procedure with milk and focus on the motion of the fat globules.

Part B: Diffusion

Introduction

In the previous activity on Brownian motion, you observed the chaotic motion of particles from ink or milk dissolved in water, which was a mixture. But how does Brownian motion play a role when two substances are mixed together? Imagine a substance dissolving in a solvent like water. The particles of the substance would move sporadically into the water, increasingly spreading out as they move farther from their source. In other words, the particles move from a region of higher concentration into one of lower concentration. This process is known as *diffusion* and is an important transport process in cells.

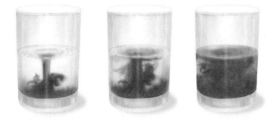

To envision this process, imagine you have a bird's-eye view of a packed festival with people moving randomly through the crowd. The police are notified that a dangerous suspect is in attendance, but they do not know where he is. A van full of police in black uniforms moves into the middle of the crowd, then the doors open and the police officers spread out in all directions.

To investigate diffusion occurring at the molecular level, conduct the following experiment.

Materials

Petri dishes with agar medium
0.1 M methylene blue solution
0.1 M potassium permanganate solution
100 mL beakers (2)
Ice
Hot plate
Stopwatch or timer
Medicine droppers
Ruler

Procedure

1. Review the content in your textbook related to diffusion.
2. Collect a Petri dish containing agar medium. Form two small wells in the agar about 3 cm from each side using the medicine dropper by placing the tip in the agar and sucking out a small portion of the medium.
3. Place a drop of the methylene blue solution in one well and a drop of the potassium permanganate solution in the other.
4. Every 15 minutes, record the distance from the point of origin that the outer boundary has progressed for each dye. Repeat three more times.
5. Create a plot to show the distance traveled over an hour for each dye and calculate the diffusion rate (rate = distance per minute).

The Effect of Temperature on the Rate of Diffusion

6. Place 50 mL of water in a beaker and place in on the hot plate until it is boiling.
7. Fill a 100 mL halfway with ice and add water to the 50 mL line.
8. Add one drop of methylene blue dye to the water in each beaker.
9. After 2 minutes, observe the rate of diffusion by observing the distribution of the dye in each beaker.

Part C: Osmosis

Introduction

Criminal organizations able to thrive over the long-term often do so because they operate like a business that acquires and exchanges goods. Whether the commodities being moved around are drugs, guns, or counterfeits, an infrastructure must exist for the proper transport of goods in and out of the organization's inventory and for their exchange. Because of this, a criminal organization cannot permit just anyone to become a member. Threats from rivals and undercover law enforcers are ever-present, and even the most insignificant lapse can be costly.

Similar transport processes are also vital to the cell. Along with the necessary transportation of molecules in and out of organelles and within the cytoplasm, cells are constantly exchanging goods with their environment through the acquisition of materials needed for survival and the elimination of wastes to avoid toxic states. Like criminal organization, the cell also requires security at points of entry. Molecular "bouncers" permit access only to select molecules and ions while ignoring other "bystanders," such as water. This security is maintained by the plasma membrane and the proteins embedded within it.

The following experiment will demonstrate the gross effects of water transport in and out of the cell across the plasma membrane, a process known as *osmosis*.

Materials

Fresh chicken eggs
Four 500-mL beakers
Vinegar
15% sucrose solution
30% sucrose solution
Distilled water
Balance
Spoon

Before You Begin

- *This may be a demonstration by your instructor.*
- *You may work in pairs if there are a limited number of eggs available.*
- *Use caution when working with eggs as fresh eggs may contain salmonella.*
- *If there is not enough time to dissolve the eggshells, it is possible to conduct this experiment using the semi-permeable membrane of the egg yolk, which requires separating the yolk from the egg white and handling it carefully during the rest of the experiment.*

Procedure

1. Review the content in your textbook related to osmosis.
2. When permitted, molecules in a substance will diffuse throughout a solution to produce an even distribution. However, some materials act as a molecular sieve, discriminating between molecules by size or by their charge, and allowing only certain molecules to pass. Plasma membranes behave this way to prevent unwanted molecules from leeching into the cell. Because of this, the plasma membrane is referred to as a *selectively permeable membrane* and the diffusion of water through one of these types of membranes is called *osmosis*.
3. To begin your investigation of osmosis, immerse two fresh eggs into separate beakers containing vinegar and allow them to sit for approximately one day or until the eggshells are completely dissolved.
4. The thin film that surrounds an egg white is a selectively permeable membrane and the eggshell must be dissolved to study the membrane directly. Although thicker than the phospholipid bilayer that makes up the plasma membrane of a cell, this film allows for the passage of water through a passive transport process.
5. Be sure to handle the eggs only with a spoon for the rest of the experiment.
6. Carefully remove the eggs from solution, rinse and dry them gently, and weigh each separately using a balance. This is the initial weight.
7. Place one egg into a 15% sucrose solution and the other into a 30% sucrose solution. These are hypertonic solutions because there is a higher concentration of solute (sucrose) in the environment than in the egg.
8. After 15 minutes, carefully remove the eggs from the solutions, rinse and dry them gently, and weigh each separately using a balance. Place them back into their respective solutions after weighing them.
9. Repeat steps 3-4 three more times and record your results.

10. Place the eggs into separate beakers of distilled water. This is a hypotonic solution because there is a lower concentration of solutes in the environment than in the egg.

11. After 15 minutes, carefully remove the eggs from solution, rinse and dry them gently, and weigh each separately using a balance. Place them back into their respective solutions after weighing them.

12. Repeat steps 6-7 three more times and record your results.

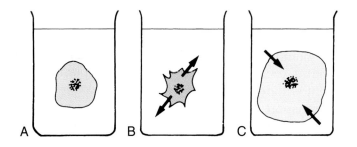

A, a cell in isotonic solution. *B*, a cell in hypertonic solution. *C*, a cell in hypotonic solution. The arrows show direction of net osmosis.

Lab Report for 3.3

Section A. Activities for Transport in the Cell

Part A: Brownian Motion

Observations

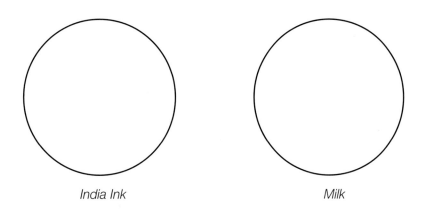

India Ink   Milk

1.   Compare your observations of the India ink and milk solutions.

2.   Which components are demonstrating Brownian motion: the globules in India ink and milk, water molecules, or both? Explain your answer.

3.   Imagine if the globule sizes were much larger than what you observed. How would their motion be different?

Part B: Diffusion

Observations

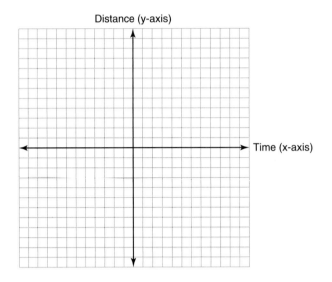

Distance (y-axis)

Time (x-axis)

1. The agar in the Petri dish contains water. During the experiment, are water molecules experiencing diffusion? Explain your answer.

2. What factors might play a role in the dyes having different diffusion rates?

3. How does temperature affect the rate of diffusion?

Part C: Osmosis

Observations

1. A cell is placed in a hypertonic solution. Which direction will water flow? What effect will that have on the cell? Explain your answer.

2. In the following figure, assess the state of the red blood cells and label each cell as hypotonic, isotonic, or hypertonic.

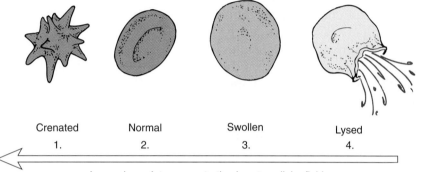

Crenated	Normal	Swollen	Lysed
1.	2.	3.	4.

Increasing solute concentration in extracellular fluid

1.	3.
2.	4.

Section B. Assessments

1. T/F   A solvent's molecules do not undergo diffusion when a solute is placed in the solvent.
2. A blood cell is placed in a hypotonic solution. What would you expect to observe?
    a. The blood cell will become larger.
    b. The blood cell will shrink.
    c. The blood cell will explode.
    d. The blood cell will stay the same size.
3. If a 15% glucose solution were separated from a 30% glucose solution by a membrane that was permeable to both water and glucose:
    a. glucose would move from the 15% solution to the 30% solution.
    b. water would move from the 15% solution to the 30% solution.
    c. the movement of glucose between the two solutions would be equal.
    d. water would move from the 30% solution to the 15% solution.

Section C. Critical Thinking Problems

Part A: Brownian Motion

1. In studying transport processes in the cell, why is it important to take Brownian motion into account?

2. What are some advantages and disadvantages of Brownian motion occurring inside the cell in light of the numerous cellular processes going on?

Part B: Diffusion

1. How would the rate of diffusion change if the agar was 10° C warmer? Explain your answer.

2. When molecules diffuse, they move from a higher concentration to a lower one, which is known as a *concentration gradient*. This concentration gradient is even more severe when a membrane is involved. Molecules can also move across a membrane because of pressure; that is, they move from an area of higher pressure to lower pressure.

   What is a common laboratory technique that takes advantage of this pressure gradient? Explain your answer.

Part C: Osmosis

1. How does a tea bag demonstrate osmosis?

2. Why can't we drink seawater?

Activity #4 — Life Cycle of the Cell

Materials

Models of mitosis
Slides of animal cell mitosis (preferably whitefish)
Slides of onion root tip
Microscope

Introduction

The life of a cell is marked by two major events: cellular division, or mitosis, and death, which is known as *apoptosis*. While the reasons for and mechanisms involved with cellular death are a subject of much current research, cellular division has been studied since Walther Flemming first reported it in 1878. Mitosis occurs because when it grows, a cell's volume increases at a faster rate than its surface. Without cellular division, a cell would experience the same outcome that a balloon inflated with too much air does: the strain at the surface would be too great and it would rupture. By dividing, the cell alleviates its growth problem while duplicating itself.

In this exercise, you will familiarize yourself with the various stages of the cell cycle as well as the cellular structures that play key roles in splitting the cell in half.

Procedure

1. Review the content in your textbook related to the cell cycle.
2. Examine both the models and the slides of each step in the cell cycle and sketch your observation in your lab report. Be sure to interpret what you are viewing in terms of the cellular structures involved and the exact stage being depicted. Knowing what each stage looks like and how it fits into the life cycle should be your focus.

Lab Report for 3.4

Section A. Activities for Life Cycle of the Cell

Using the slides you have been provided, complete the following chart by sketching in your observations of the appropriate phase in mitosis below.

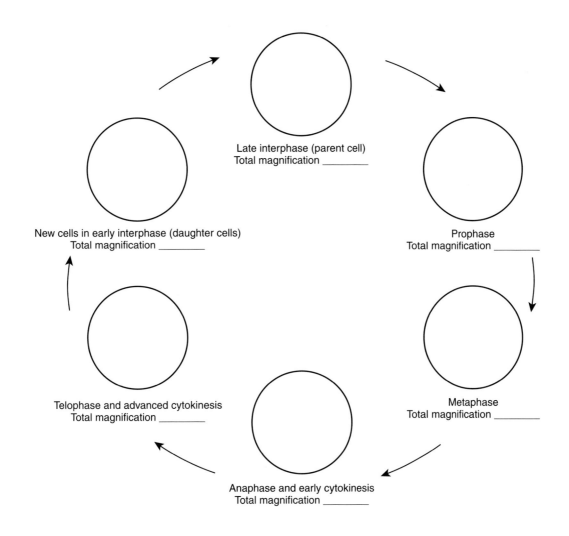

Late interphase (parent cell)
Total magnification _____

Prophase
Total magnification _____

Metaphase
Total magnification _____

Anaphase and early cytokinesis
Total magnification _____

Telophase and advanced cytokinesis
Total magnification _____

New cells in early interphase (daughter cells)
Total magnification _____

Section B. Assessments

1. T/F   A cell in interphase is not actively involved in cell division.

2. Match the phase of mitosis with each description of the event during that phase.

a.	anaphase	_____	Chromosomes align in the middle of the cell
b.	interphase	_____	DNA replication occurs
c.	metaphase	_____	The nuclear envelope reforms around daughter nuclei
d.	prophase	_____	Chromatin condenses into chromosomes and becomes visible
e.	telophase	_____	Chromosomes are pulled to opposite poles of the cell

Section C. Critical Thinking Problem

1. Why is it important to control how often mitosis is occurring in a group of cells?

Exercise 4

Tissues: Organization and Classification

Lesson Overview

Activity #1: Epithelial Tissues
Activity #2: Connective Tissues
Activity #3: Muscle and Nervous Tissues

Overview

If people lived in a state of anarchy where laws weren't enforced, criminals wouldn't exist simply because everything would be permitted. The police exist to protect law-abiding citizens from the consequences of criminal activity by identifying and incarcerating those responsible. These three groups—law enforcers, law abiders, and lawbreakers—are intertwined in society.

In the body, tissues are organizations of cells of particular types, and in a sense, cells within tissues comply with certain "laws" that give the cells uniformity and specific characteristics. After all, cellular anarchy would prevent any multicellular eukaryote from existing. Various mechanisms exist to enforce these laws to ensure that any lawbreaking cells are quickly repaired or disposed of. However, just as criminal organizations are able to elude police and thrive within society, certain cells circumvent cellular law and become cancerous.

In our study of tissues, we will systematically investigate the characteristic features of epithelial, connective, muscle and nervous tissue and classify them according to these features.

Epithelial tissue lines
surfaces in the body

Muscle tissue is made
up of fibers that contract

Bone and cartilage
are connective
tissues made up of
cells in hard or stiff
extracellular matrix

Cartilage

Bone

Blood is a connective tissue made
up of cells in a liquid matrix

Protein
fibers

Soft
extracellular
matrix

Cells

Loose connective tissue acts
as padding under skin and
elsewhere

Nervous tissue consists of cells with
projections that transmit electrical
signals

Activity #1 — Epithelial Tissues

Introduction

Epithelial tissue covers the surfaces and cavities within the body and can also form glands. As a covering, it always has one side exposed, just as cellophane has one side facing outward regardless of what it is wrapped around. The tissue itself is avascular and has little intercellular space, with cells densely packed together.

Materials

Slides of epithelial tissue, with and without labels including stratified epithelium, simple cuboidal epithelium, columnar epithelium, and pseudostratified epithelium

Microscope

Procedure

1. Review the content from your textbook related to epithelial tissues.
2. Micrographs of epithelial tissue are provided for reference in Figure 4.2, while characteristic features of epithelial cells are shown in Figure 4.3. Additionally, the classification scheme to follow in the text is in the form of a chart in Figure 4.4.
3. Epithelial tissue is classified structurally by determining the number of cell layers within a sheet: simple has one layer, stratified has more than one layer, and pseudostratified has only one layer but gives the illusion of having more than one because of the ways the cells are packed within the layer.
4. To further classify simple and striated epithelial tissue, examine the layer of cells on the tissue's open surface and identify them as either squamous, cuboidal, columnar, or transitional.
5. Both pseudostratified and simple columnar epithelial cells can be further categorized as ciliated or nonciliated, depending on whether cilia are present.
6. Finally, stratified squamous tissue can be further differentiated as keratinized or nonkeratinized, depending on whether it contains keratin, which is a tough, fibrous protein.
7. Use the microscope to make observations about the epithelial tissue on the labeled slides provided and make sketches of each tissue type in your lab report. You will need to draw specific features of these tissues, such as size, shape, and organization of the cells, in order to differentiate each type.
8. Using the classification scheme in Figure 4.4, sketch the epithelial tissue from each of the three unknown slides (slides A, B, and C) provided by your instructor in your lab report and correctly identify them.

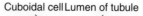

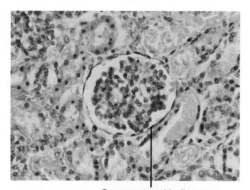

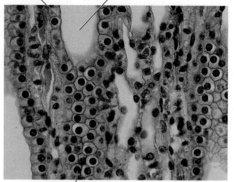

Squamous epithelium

Cell nuclei

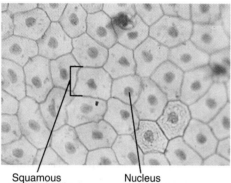

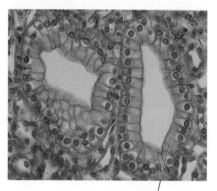

Squamous epithelial cell

Nucleus

Columnar cells

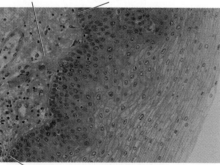

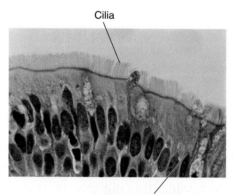

Dermis   Basement membrane

Cilia

Basal cell layer

Pseudostratified cells

Keratin layer

Basement membrane

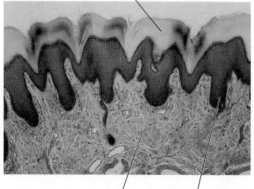

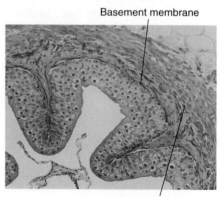

Dermis   Basement membrane

Connective tissue

Figure 4.2

Cell shapes

Squamous

Cuboidal

Columnar

Simple

(Simple squamous)

(Simple cuboidal)

(Simple columnar)

Cilia

Basement membrane

Connective tissue

(Pseudostratified)

Stratified

(Stratified squamous)

(Transitional, relaxed)

(Transitional, stretched)

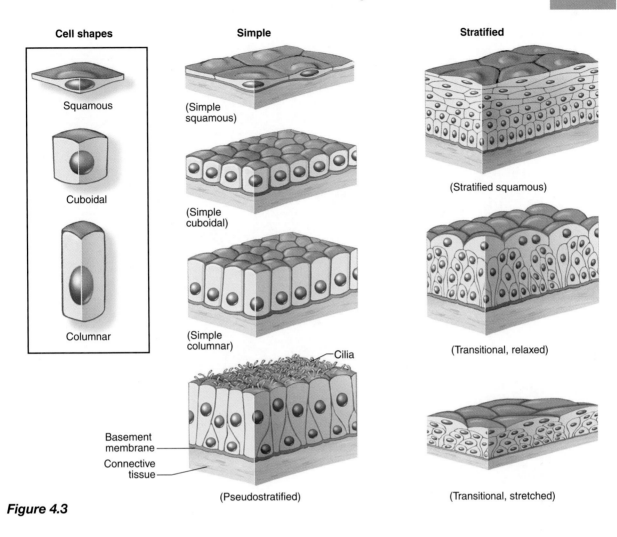

Figure 4.3

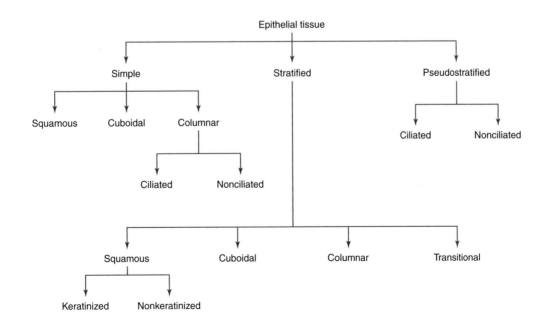

Epithelial tissue

Simple

Squamous   Cuboidal   Columnar

Ciliated   Nonciliated

Stratified

Squamous   Cuboidal   Columnar   Transitional

Keratinized   Nonkeratinized

Pseudostratified

Ciliated   Nonciliated

Figure 4.4

Lab Report for 4.1

Section A. Activities for Epithelial Tissues

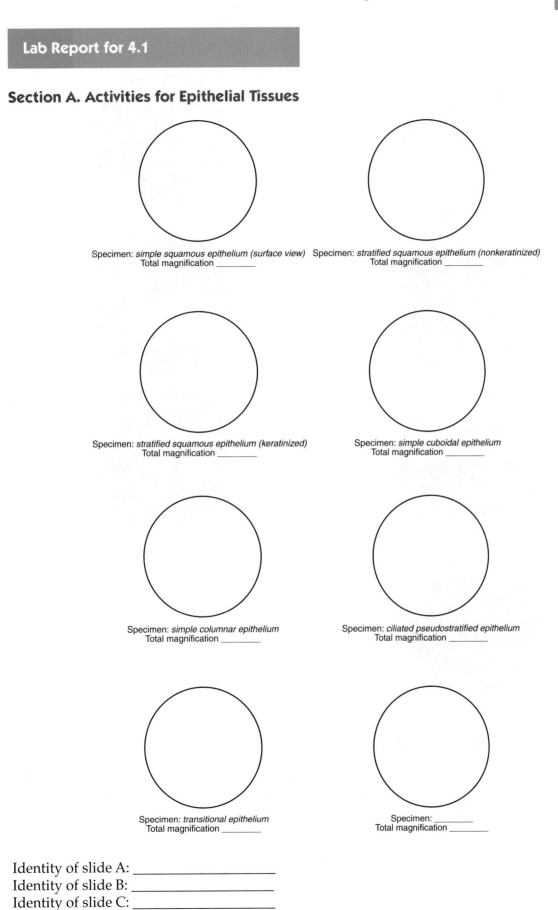

Specimen: *simple squamous epithelium (surface view)*
Total magnification _____

Specimen: *stratified squamous epithelium (nonkeratinized)*
Total magnification _____

Specimen: *stratified squamous epithelium (keratinized)*
Total magnification _____

Specimen: *simple cuboidal epithelium*
Total magnification _____

Specimen: *simple columnar epithelium*
Total magnification _____

Specimen: *ciliated pseudostratified epithelium*
Total magnification _____

Specimen: *transitional epithelium*
Total magnification _____

Specimen: _____
Total magnification _____

Identity of slide A: _____
Identity of slide B: _____
Identity of slide C: _____

Identify each type of tissue.

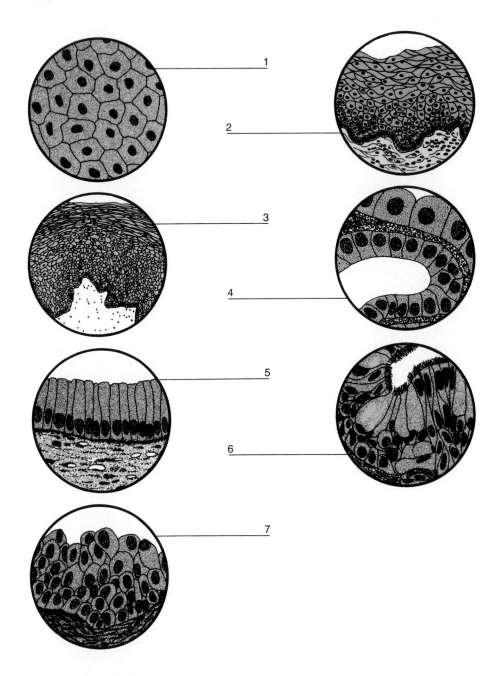

Section B. Critical Thinking Problem

1. The Introduction drew a comparison between epithelial tissue and cellophane wrap. Consider the features of both: depending on what they are being used for, how similar are their properties, such as permeability?

Activity #2 — Connective Tissues

Introduction

If law is what holds civilization together, connective tissue is the glue of the body, holding its parts together and providing structural support. This is also true of blood, which is a connective tissue, in the sense that it connects tissues throughout the body through the dynamic transport of nutrients. Unlike epithelial tissue, connective tissues contain a significant amount of nonliving components within their extracellular matrix. The primary role of connective tissue is for support, and this can be in the form of:

- gross structural support, as is the case with bones
- bridging support, such as tendons and ligaments that connect tissues (hence, the name of the tissue type)
- mechanical support, such as adipose tissue, that along with storing energy in the form of fat, provides cushioning for such things as the system of ducts in the breast

Materials

Slides of connective tissue, with and without labels including hyaline cartilage, dense fibrous connective tissue such as a tendon, adipose tissue, blood smear, compact bone, and loose areolar tissue
Microscope

Procedure

1. Review the content from your textbook related to connective tissues.
2. Micrographs of connective tissue are provided in Figure 4.6 for reference, while characteristic features of connective cells are shown in Figure 4.7. The classification scheme to follow in the text is in the form of a chart in Figure 4.8.

3. Connective tissue is classified by characterizing the basic type of matrix present, whether it is a protein matrix, a protein/ground substance matrix, or a fluid matrix.
4. Connective tissue with a protein matrix contains fibrous proteins, such as collagen, and can be further separated into adipose, also called *fat* tissue, or fibrous tissue, of which there are three types categorized by the density of the protein fibers: loose, reticular (containing collagen), and dense (which can be regular or irregular, depending on the organization of the fibers).
5. Extracellular materials with a protein/ground substance matrix contain some fibrous proteins mixed with other substances, such as cartilage or bone. Cartilage comes in three forms: hyaline cartilage (which contains some collagen), fibrocartilage (containing a large amount of collagen), and elastic cartilage that has the flexible elastin proteins. Bone, on the other hand, is either compact with large, dense areas of matrix, or spongy (cancellous) with thin portions of hard bone.
6. Connective tissue with a fluid matrix is either blood or hematopoietic tissue, which is also known as *red bone marrow*.
7. Use the microscope to make observations about the connective tissue on the labeled slides provided and make sketches of each tissue type in your lab report. You will need to draw specific features of these tissues, such as size, shape, and organization of the cells, in order to differentiate each type.
8. Using the classification scheme in Figure 4.8, sketch the connective tissue from each of the three unknown slides (slides D, E, and F) provided by your instructor in your lab report and correctly identify the kind of epithelial tissue it is.

Elastin fibers

Nuclei of adipocyte Fat (lipid) storage area

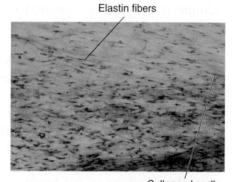

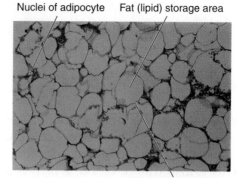

Collagen bundle

Plasma membrane

Reticular fibers

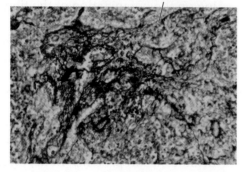

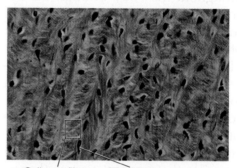

Collagen fibers Fibroblast

Collagen fibers Fibroblast

Cartilaginous matrix Perichondrium

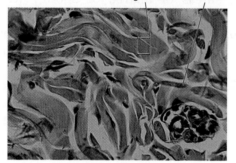

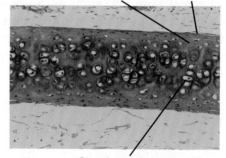

Chondrocyte in lacuna

Figure 4.6

Collagen fiber matrix

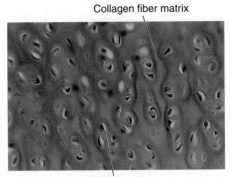

Cells in lacuna

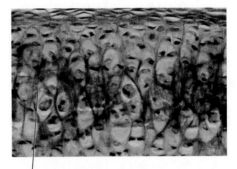

Elastin fibers

Osteon

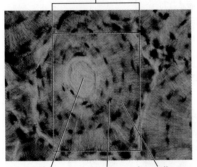

Haversian canal   Lacuna   Lamellae

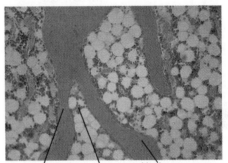

Matrix   Bone marrow   Nucleus

Large lymphocyte   Erythrocyte

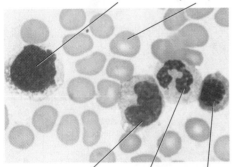

Monocyte   Neutrophil   Lymphocyte

Figure 4.6 (con't.)

TISSUE	LOCATION	FUNCTION
Fibrous		
Loose (areolar)	Between other tissues and organs Superficial fascia	Connection Connection
Adipose (fat)	Under skin Padding at various points	Protection Insulation Support Reserve food
Reticular	Inner framework of spleen, lymph nodes, bone marrow Filtration	Support
Dense Fibrous		
Irregular	Deep fascia Dermis Scars Capsule of kidney, etc.	Connection Support
Regular Collagenous	Tendons Ligaments Aponeuroses	Flexible but strong connection
Elastic	Walls of some arteries	Flexible, elastic support

TISSUE	LOCATION	FUNCTION
Bone		
Compact bone	Skeleton (outer shell of bones)	Support Protection Calcium reservoir
Cancellous (spongy) bone	Skeleton (inside bones)	Support Provides framework for blood production
Cartilage		
Hyaline	Part of nasal septum Covering articular surfaces of bones Larynx Rings in trachea and bronchi	Firm but flexible support
Fibrocartilage	Disks between vertebrae Pubic symphysis	
Elastic	External ear Eustachian or auditory tube	
Blood		
	In the blood vessels	Transportation Protection

Figure 4.7

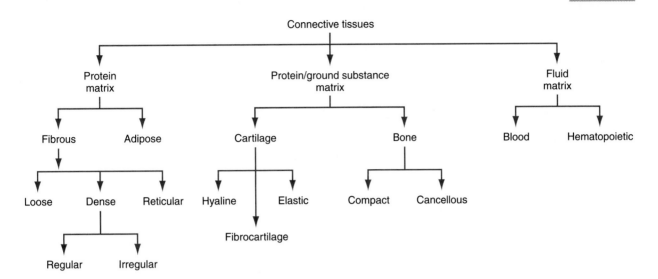

Figure 4.8

Lab Report for 4.2

Section A. Activities for Connective Tissues

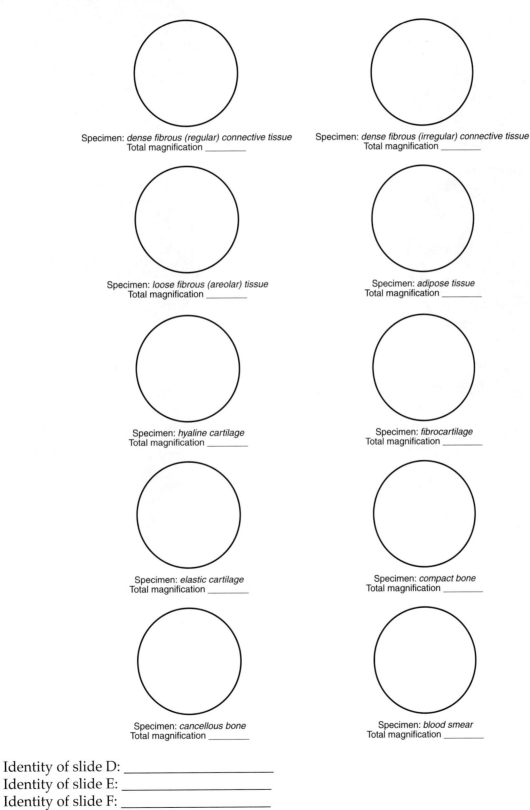

Specimen: *dense fibrous (regular) connective tissue*
Total magnification _____

Specimen: *dense fibrous (irregular) connective tissue*
Total magnification _____

Specimen: *loose fibrous (areolar) tissue*
Total magnification _____

Specimen: *adipose tissue*
Total magnification _____

Specimen: *hyaline cartilage*
Total magnification _____

Specimen: *fibrocartilage*
Total magnification _____

Specimen: *elastic cartilage*
Total magnification _____

Specimen: *compact bone*
Total magnification _____

Specimen: *cancellous bone*
Total magnification _____

Specimen: *blood smear*
Total magnification _____

Identity of slide D: _____

Identity of slide E: _____

Identity of slide F: _____

Identify each type of connective tissue.

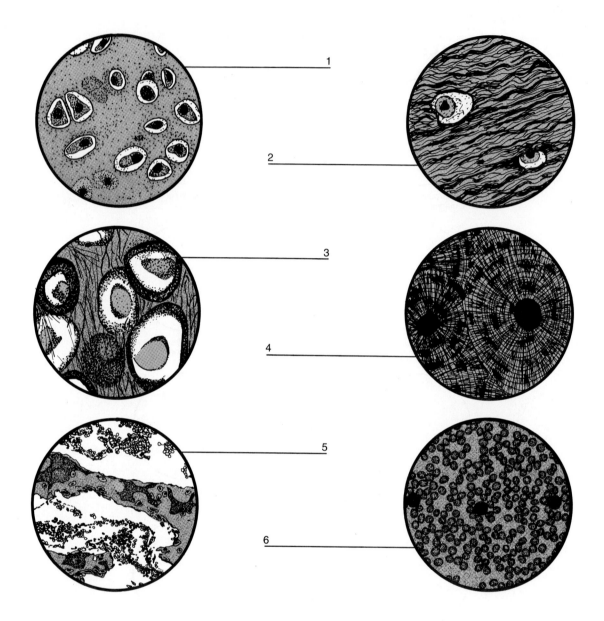

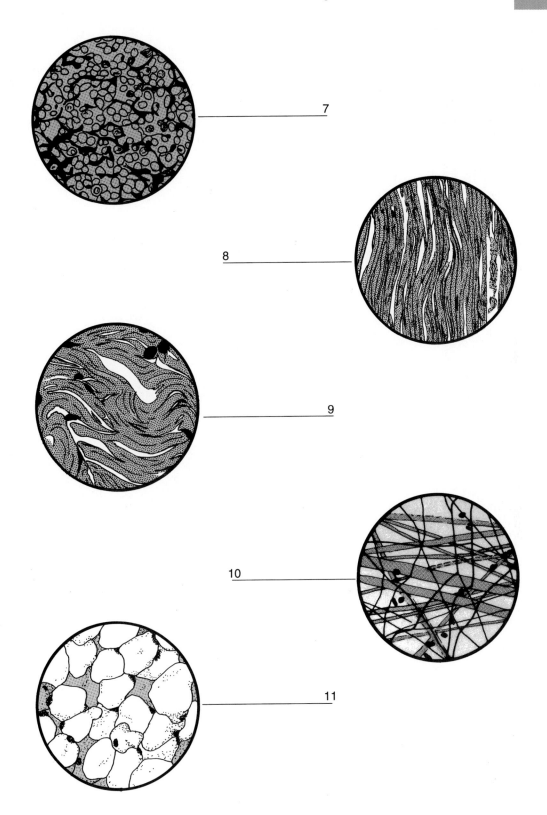

Section B. Critical Thinking Problem

1. When a body or human remains are discovered at a crime scene, forensic pathologists determine the cause of death based on the state of the tissues and the various injuries to them. This is true whether death occurred recently or if the pathologist has nothing but skeletal remains to examine. What types of connective tissues, and their properties, might a pathologist find the most helpful in determining the nature of a crime? Which would be the least helpful? Explain your answers.

Activity #3 — Muscle and Nervous Tissues

Introduction

Muscle tissue contracts in response to an electrical stimulus, stretches when pulling forces are applied to it, and returns to its original shape. These characteristics will ultimately allow for movement in the human body, whether voluntary, as in skeletal muscle, or involuntary, as occurs in cardiac and smooth muscle.

Nervous tissue is by far the most straightforward to identify, simply because there are only two types of cells known: neurons and neuroglia. Yet neurons are unusual among cells because they contain a central body, which houses the nucleus, and extensive branching into processes, one of which can extend to lengths up to 1 m. These cells are both the receivers and conductors of electrical signals. Their amazing functionality comes from their role in the network of the nervous system. While there are many types of neuroglia, their primary function is to surround neurons for support.

Materials

Slides of muscle and nervous tissue, with and without labels
Microscope

Procedure

1. Review the content from your textbook related to muscle and nervous tissues.
2. Micrographs of muscle and nervous tissue are provided for reference in Figure 4.10, while characteristic features of muscle and nervous cells are shown in Figure 4.11.
3. The elongated, multinucleate cells of skeletal muscle tissue, named so because they are responsible for the voluntary motion of the skeleton, are organized into distinct striations running in parallel that provide coordinated contraction.
4. Cardiac muscle tissue, found only in the walls of the heart, contain non-nucleate cells that are branched and contain striations that are connected by intercalated discs.
5. Smooth muscle tissue is found within internal structures that act as containers, such as the stomach, arteries, and veins, and the lungs, and are noteworthy because they consist of layers that lack striations, providing for fuller ranges of motion.
6. Use the microscope to make observations about the muscle and nervous tissue on the labeled slides provided and make sketches of each tissue type in your lab report. You will need to identify characteristic features of these tissues, such as size, shape, and organization of the cells, which will allow you to differentiate each type.
7. Sketch the muscle and nervous tissue from each of the three unknown slides (slides G, H, and I) provided by your instructor in your lab report and correctly identify them.

Striations

Nuclei

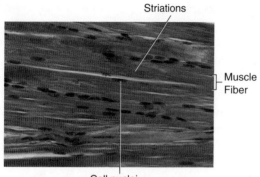

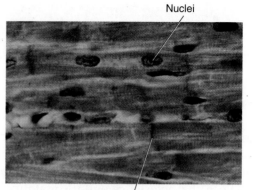

Muscle Fiber

Cell nuclei

Intercalated disks

Smooth muscle cell

Soma (cell body)   Axon

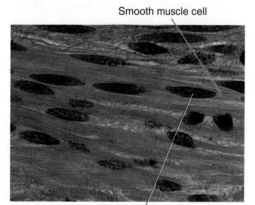

Nuclei

Dendrite

Figure 4.10

TISSUE	LOCATION	FUNCTION
Muscle		
Skeletal (striated voluntary)	Muscles that attach to bones Extrinsic eyeball muscles Upper third of the esophagus	Movement of bones Eye movements First part of swallowing
Smooth (nonstriated, involuntary, or visceral)	In the walls of tubular viscera of the digestive, respiratory, and genitourinary tracts In the walls of blood vessels and large lymphatic vessels In the ducts of glands Intrinsic eye muscles (iris and ciliary body) Arrector muscles of hairs	Movement of substances along the respective tracts Change diameter of blood vessels, thereby aiding in regulation of blood pressure Movement of substances along ducts Change diameter of pupils and shape of the lens Erection of hairs (gooseflesh)
Cardiac (striated involuntary)	Wall of the heart	Contraction of the heart
Nervous		
	Brain Spinal cord Nerves	Excitability Conduction

Figure 4.11

Lab Report for 4.3

Section A. Activities for Muscle and Nervous Tissues

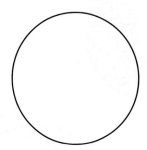

Specimen: *skeletal muscle*
Total magnification _____

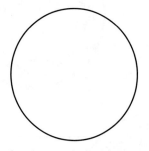

Specimen: *cardiac muscle*
Total magnification _____

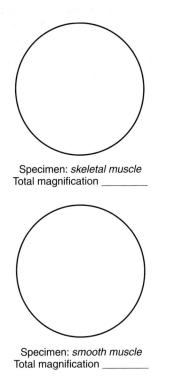

Specimen: *smooth muscle*
Total magnification _____

Specimen: *spinal cord smear*
Total magnification _____

Identity of slide G: _____
Identity of slide H: _____
Identity of slide I: _____

Identify each type of tissue.

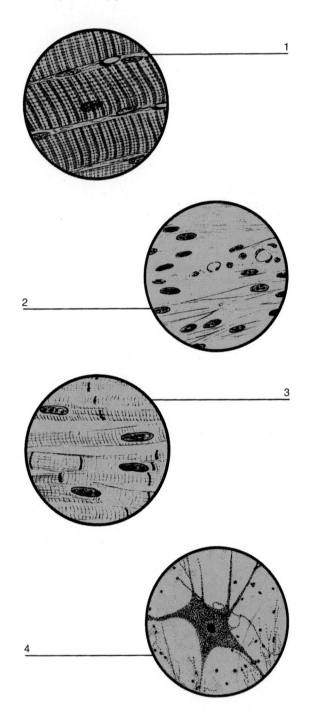

1 _____

2 _____

3 _____

4 _____

Section B. Critical Thinking Problems

1. Within the heart, a specialized area of cardiac muscle tissue has cells that can contract on their own between 60-100 contractions per minute without an impulse from the nervous system. Why would this be advantageous to cardiac muscle tissue, but not to skeletal or smooth muscle tissue?

2. What structural aspect of neurons suggests that they function within a network?

Unit 2

Support and Movement

"And a lean, silent figure slowly fades into the gathering darkness, aware at last that in this world, with great power there must also come—great responsibility."

- Stan Lee, from the first of Spider-Man in *Amazing Fantasy #15*, 1962

What makes a superhero super?

Superheroes are super for a variety of reasons. For some, their superiority is a birthright, their unique genetics imbuing them with powers beyond those of mere mortals. Wonder Woman, for instance, isn't human; she is the youngest of the mythological Amazons. Some superheroes are born with mutations to their otherwise average human genetics, giving them unusual powers, as is the case with the X-Men.

For some superheroes, and for many villains, an extreme event transforms their bodies into super physiques. Peter Parker succumbed to the effects of a radioactive spider bite to become Spider-Man. Another young man, deemed unfit to serve by the Army, is given a super-soldier serum and transformed into the pinnacle of human potential — Captain America.

In rare cases, humans are able to attain the status of superhero through a combination of genius-level intellects, extreme training and a wealth of technological gadgets. Both Batman and Iron Man have human DNA — presumably mutation-free and uncompromised — and yet they achieve incredible, superhuman feats through their physical and mental prowess and sheer will.

By reflecting on superhero abilities and comparing them to those of the average citizen, we can gain a sense of the normal range of musculoskeletal form and function and an appreciation of the "super-ness" of costumed avengers.

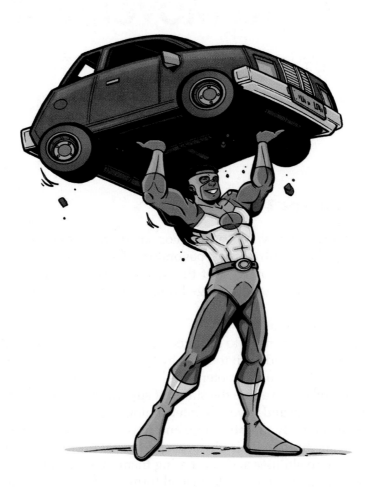

Exercise 5
The Musculoskeletal System

Lesson Overview

Activity #1: Organization of the Skeletal System
Activity #2: Organization of the Muscular System

Overview

Artists who create superheroes strive to capture human-like qualities related to the appearance of power, but not necessarily the logistics of it. Comic book artists study human anatomy but rarely physiology. After all, superheroes are exaggerations of the physical attributes of humans, such as shape, musculature, stature, and proportionality, all of which relate to the musculoskeletal system.

The musculoskeletal system is responsible for both the motion and support of the body, while also producing the shape of the human form. These two systems are interdependent and understanding the organization of each is essential to the appreciation of the other.

We will begin our investigation with separate overviews of the skeletal and muscular system to gain a sense of how each contributes to support and motion. In later exercises, each system will be investigated in depth, and finally, we will return to the musculoskeletal system as a whole in order to study surface anatomy and range of motion.

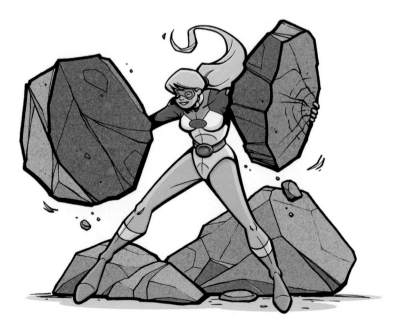

Activity #1 — Organization of the Skeletal System

Introduction

The human body contains over 200 bones that make up the skeleton. It serves as the support for everything that is attached to or contained by it. Additionally, it is a storehouse of minerals and the body's manufacturing site for the red blood cells that transport oxygen and white blood cells of the immune system. The skeletal system, traditionally divided into the axial and appendicular skeletons, determines the shape, stature, and size of both humans and superheroes. In order to appreciate its role, we begin with a general sense of the organization of the skeletal system.

Materials

Model of the skeletal system
Textbook

Procedure

1. Review content in your textbook related to the organization of the skeleton.
2. Since ancient Greek anatomists began naming the structures of the body, anatomical structures have been given terms that refer to their location, direction, size, appearance, function, discoverer, relation to other vital structures, or a combination of these, depending on the degree of accuracy required and/or the tradition of medicine.

   As you learn the names of the bones, you may find yourself at this early stage memorizing terms with little understanding of why the bone is given a particular name. Over time, as you continue to learn more about the body, the names will likely make more sense. Because bones, as well as the rest of the structures in the body, are named for a variety of reasons, names cannot be taught systematically but must be learned more like a native language — first imitation, then explanation.

3. Identify the major parts of the skeleton in an idealized human body according to the following table:

4. It may be helpful to compare the analogous bones of the upper and lower extremities, both for the sake of terminology and functional understanding.

BONES OF THE SKELETON (206 TOTAL)*	
PART OF BODY	**NAME OF BONE**
Axial Skeleton (80 Bones Total)	
Skull (28 bones total)	
Cranium (8 bones)	Frontal (1) Parietal (2) Temporal (2) Occipital (1) Sphenoid (1) Ethmoid (1)
Face (14 bones)	Nasal (2) Maxillary (2) Zygomatic (malar) (2) Mandible (1) Lacrimal (2) Palatine (2) Inferior nasal conchae (turbinates) (2) Vomer (1)
Ear bones (6 bones)	Malleus (hammer) (2) Incus (anvil) (2) Stapes (stirrup) (2)
Hyoid bone (1)	
Spinal column (26 bones total)	Cervical vertebrae (7) Thoracic vertebrae (12) Lumbar vertebrae (5) Sacrum (1) Coccyx (1)
Sternum and ribs (25 bones total)	Sternum (1) True ribs (14) False ribs (10)
Appendicular Skeleton (126 Bones Total)	
Upper extremities (including shoulder girdle) (64 bones total)	Clavicle (2) Scapula (2) Humerus (2) Radius (2) Ulna (2) Carpal bones (16) Metacarpal bones (10) Phalanges (28)
Lower extremities (including hip girdle) (62 bones total)	Innominate (2) Fibula (2) Femur (2) Patella (2) Tibia (2) Tarsal bones (14) Metatarsal bones (10) Phalanges (28)

*An inconstant number of small, flat, round bones known as *sesamoid bones* (because of their resemblance to sesame seeds) are found in various tendons in which considerable pressure develops. Because the number of these bones varies greatly between individuals, only two of them, the patellae, have been counted among the 206 bones of the body. Generally, two of them can be found in each thumb (in the flexor tendon near the metacarpophalangeal and interphalangeal joints) and great toe, plus several others in the upper and lower extremities. *Sutural bones (wormian bones),* the small islets of bone frequently found in some of the cranial sutures, have not been counted in this list of 206 bones because of their variable occurrence.

Lab Report for 5.1

Section A. Activities for Organization of the Skeletal System

1. Identify the major bones in the following charts (see also next page):

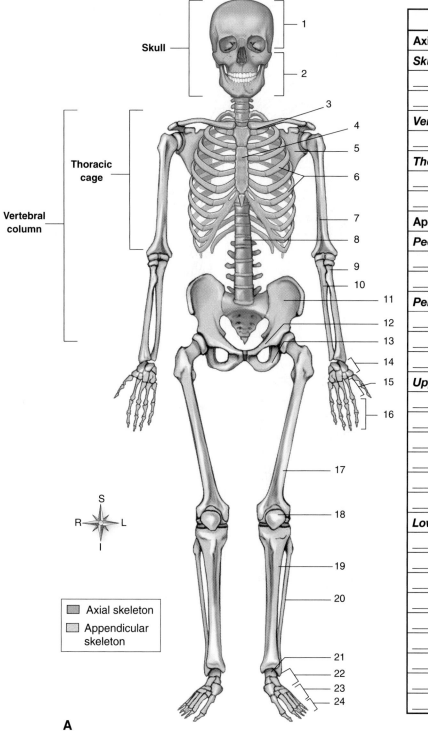

Relevant Terms
Axial Skeleton
Skull
_____ Cranium
_____ Facial bones
Vertebral Column
_____ Vertebrae
Thoracic Cage
_____ Ribs
_____ Sternum
Appendicular Skeleton
Pectoral Girdle
_____ Clavicle
_____ Scapula
Pelvic Girdle
_____ Ilium
_____ Ischium
_____ Pubis
Upper Extremity
_____ Carpals
_____ Humerus
_____ Metacarpals
_____ Phalanges
_____ Radius
_____ Ulna
Lower Extremity
_____ Calcaneus
_____ Femur
_____ Fibula
_____ Metatarsals
_____ Patella
_____ Phalanges
_____ Talus
_____ Tarsals
_____ Tibia

A

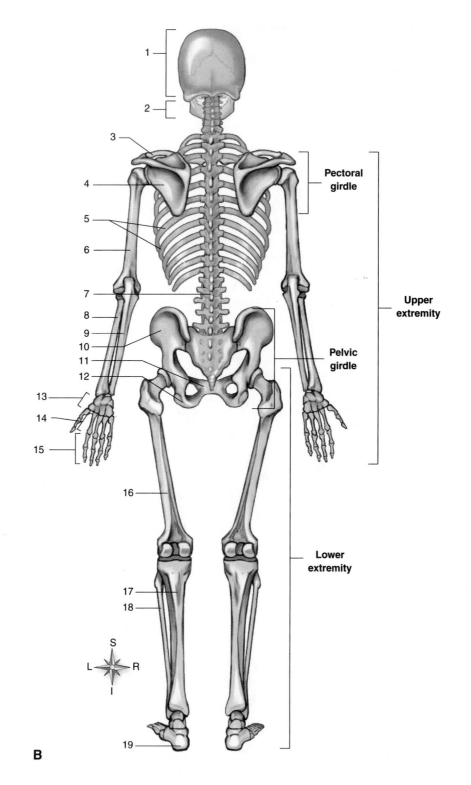

1

2

3

4

5

6

7

8

9

10

11

12

13

14

15

16

17

18

19

Pectoral girdle

Upper extremity

Pelvic girdle

Lower extremity

S

L R

I

B

Section B. Assessments

1. T/F   The axial skeleton contains fewer bones than the appendicular skeleton.
2. T/F   Just like bones in a graveyard, bones inside a person are not alive.
3. Which of the following is NOT a function of the skeletal system?
   a. blood cell production
   b. motion
   c. storage of calcium
   d. all of the above are skeletal system functions
4. All of the following bones are part of the appendicular skeleton EXCEPT:
   a. hyoid bone.
   b. ulna.
   c. humerus.
   d. tibia.
5. Match the location or description to each bone below.
   a. femur   _____ fingers and toes
   b. humerus   _____ foot
   c. ulna   _____ kneecap
   d. fibula   _____ lower arm
   e. mandible   _____ lower jaw
   f. metatarsals   _____ lower leg
   g. patella   _____ thigh
   h. phalanges   _____ upper arm

Section C. Critical Thinking Problems

1. Which parts of the body have the most bones? What advantage is there to having many bones in these parts as opposed to a few?

2. A typical human body is 7.5 head-lengths high, but when comic book artists draw superheroes, it is recommended that the length of the body be extended to 8.5 head-lengths. This is referred to as a "heroic" figure and is accomplished by extending the proportionate lengths of the chest and legs. How would changing these proportions of the head to the rest of the body cause the appearance of a figure to seem heroic?

3. The video game and the subsequent film *Mortal Combat* included Goro, a powerful creature that had four arms, the two additional arms attached to the lower ribcage. What anatomical and functional issues might arise if two arms were attached at this point? Is there a way that two additional arms could be attached to the human skeleton and have the same support and muscle attachments as the upper extremities?

Activity #2 — Organization of the Muscular System

Introduction

Superheroes are all about action. Batman, for instance, may concoct clever plans in his bat cave, use advanced technology to spy on the illegal activities of archnemeses, and brood about bringing them to justice *ad nauseam*, but he isn't really a superhero until he does more than mental gymnastics. Although strategy, teamwork, and quick thinking all play a part in the success of superhero efforts, in the end it often comes down to physical strength to save the day.

Muscles, like superheroes, have jobs to do. Specifically, they must generate the three kinds of large-scale motion that the body requires: the circulation of blood, the passage of food, and the movement of the skeleton. Though cardiac muscle contracts on its own as it regulates heart contractions, it does so sporadically. In its own way, it's a lot like the Incredible Hulk: powerful but effective only when controlled. Smooth muscle serves multiple functions in the body when involuntary motion is required, such as helping food move through the intestines and supporting blood transport in the circulatory system. It serves its function in the background, quietly performing its job with little fanfare, much like the less popular, one-dimensional superheroes of the X-Men. Skeletal muscle makes sudden action possible by moving the bones around, thereby grabbing the spotlight. In its own way, it is the Superman of muscles.

Because the task of the more than 600 skeletal muscles is to move and support bones, the organization of the muscular system mirrors the organization of the skeletal system. Unlike the framework of the skeletal system, however, the muscular system is built up in layers, with different layers often connected to different bones to produce specific movements. Here, muscles will be classified into four groups: muscles of the head and face, the core, the upper extremities, and the lower extremities. In Exercise 3 of this Unit, we will investigate the groupings of the muscular system in greater detail.

Materials

Model of the muscular system
Textbook

Procedure

1. Review content in your textbook related to the organization of the muscles.
2. Identify the major muscles in the human body according to Figures 5.4 a and b.
3. It may be helpful to relate the analogous muscles of the upper and lower extremities, both for the sake of terminology and functional understanding.

Lab Report for 5.2

Section A. Activities for Organization of the Muscular System

1. Identify the major muscles in the following charts (see also next page):

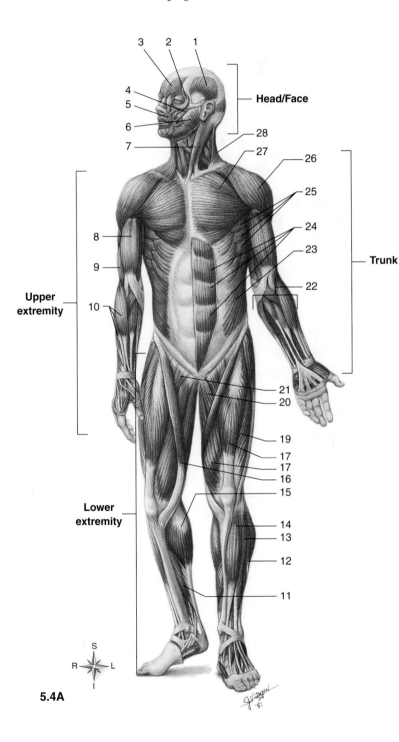

5.4A

Relevant Terms
Head/Face
_____ Masseter
_____ Occipitofrontalis
_____ Orbicularis oculi
_____ Orbicularis oculi
_____ Orbicularis oris
_____ Sternocleidomastoid
_____ Temporalis
_____ Zygomaticus
Trunk
_____ External oblique
_____ Latissimus dorsi
_____ Pectoralis major
_____ Rectus abdominis
_____ Serratus anterior
_____ Trapezius
Upper Extremity
_____ Biceps brachii
_____ Brachialis
_____ Deltoid
_____ Triceps brachii
_____ Wrist/finger extensors
_____ Wrist/finger flexors
Lower Extremity
_____ Adductor
_____ Adductor longus
_____ Biceps femoris
_____ Calcaneal (Achilles) tendon
_____ Extensor digitorum longus
_____ Fibularis longus
_____ Gastrocnemius
_____ Iliopsoas
_____ Rectus femoris
_____ Sartorius
_____ Semimembranosus
_____ Semiteninosus
_____ Soleus
_____ Tibialis anterior
_____ Vastus lateralis
_____ Vastus medialis

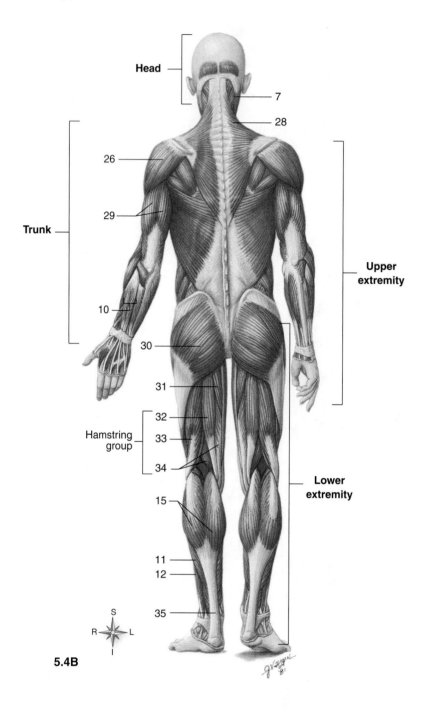

Head — 7

28

26

29

Trunk

10

30

31

32
Hamstring
group   33

34

15

11
12

S
R ⊕ L
I

35

Upper
extremity

Lower
extremity

5.4B

2. Give an example of a muscle named by: location, function, shape, fiber direction, number of heads, and points of attachment.

Section B. Assessments

1. T/F   Muscles fill in the form and contour of the body.
2. Which of the following is NOT a general function of the muscles?
   a. posture
   b. movement
   c. protection
   d. heat production
3. The muscle responsible for shrugging of shoulders is the:
   a. trapezius.
   b. pectoralis minor.
   c. deltoid.
   d. sternocleidomastoid.

Section C. Critical Thinking Problems

1. Weightlifters can increase the bulk and strength of specific muscles by isolating them during a workout. Other athletes, such as basketball players, develop muscles that work together to enhance coordination. Finally, the muscles of long-distance runners have been honed for endurance. But superheroes are often depicted as incredibly muscular, immensely strong, highly coordinated, and having great stamina. Do you think it is possible for real muscles to be all of these things without consequences?

2. Common sites for receiving an intramuscular injection are the vastus lateralis, gluteus medius, and the deltoid. Why are these good sites for these injections?

Exercise 6
The Skeletal System

Lesson Overview

Activity #1: Bone Structure and Function
   Part A: Structure of a Long Bone
   Part B: Properties of Bone
Activity #2: The Axial Skeleton
   Part A: The Skull
   Part B: Vertebral Column and Thoracic Cage
Activity #3: The Appendicular Skeleton
   Part A: Pectoral Girdle and Upper Extremities
   Part B: Pelvic Girdle and Lower Extremities
Activity #4: Joints

Overview

Both the broad-shouldered, barrel-chested, square-jawed virility of the male superhero and the Barbie-like, disproportionate, hourglass figure of the superheroine convey masculine and feminine power, respectively. These body shapes are some of the most prominent and familiar features of superheroes, to the point of being cliché. Yet underneath their costumes, skin, and muscles, superheroes have skeletal systems made of bones and joints no different than our own. Understanding how these bones connect together to form the skeleton helps us appreciate both human and superhuman anatomy.

To begin the study of the skeletal system, we will examine the structure and properties of bones. We will then systematically cover the two divisions of the skeletal system, the axial and appendicular system, and learn how individual bones organize into much larger functional parts of the body.

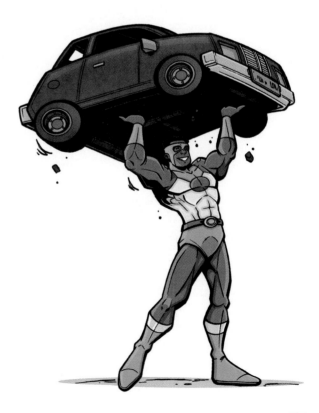

Activity #1 — Bone Structure and Function

Part A: Structure of a Long Bone

Introduction

Few superheroes have bone enhancements. An exception is Logan, commonly known as Wolverine, who has a mutation that produced bone claws, among other bodily enhancements, and a fictitious durable metal alloy called *adamantium* bonded to his entire skeleton. Human bones are often misunderstood, perhaps because we lack the X-ray vision of Supergirl to see bones as they are inside the body. As with other organs, bones are the convergence of multiple systems, containing connective, blood, and nervous tissue. Bone consists of both an organic matrix and inorganic minerals. While serving as both a support system and a protector of the softer tissues around them, bones are anchors for muscles, storehouses of minerals, and manufacturers of blood cells. Bones are more than just an underlying framework — they are an active and vital organ system.

Materials

Textbook
Disarticulated human skeleton
Articulated human skeleton (for reference)
Human long bone cut longitudinally
Microscope
Slides of compact bone, cancellous bone, and an epiphyseal plate

Procedure

1. Review content in your textbook related to bone structure.
2. Divide the bones of a disarticulated human skeleton into the four categories: long, short, flat, and irregular. Note the similarities and differences of each group.
3. Examine a long bone and locate its major features in Figure 6.2.
4. Practice using the terms for bone markings indicated in Table 6.1.
5. Examine various types of prepared bone tissue slides including compact bone, cancellous bone, and an epiphyseal plate, if available, and draw what you observe in your lab report. Be sure to relate the features of each tissue type to the overall structure or function of a long bone.

Term	Meaning
Angle	A corner
Body	The main portion of a bone
Condyle	Rounded bump; usually fits into a fossa on another bone to form a joint
Crest	Moderately raised ridge; generally a site for muscle attachement
Epicondyle	Bump near a condyle; often gives the appearance of a "bump on a bump;" for muscle attachment
Facet	Flat surface that forms a joint with another facet or flat bone
Fissure	Long, cracklike hole for blood vessels and nerves
Foramen	Round hole for vessels and nerves (*pl.*, foramina)
Fossa	Depression; often receives an articulating bone
Head	Distinct epiphysis on a long bone, separated from the shaft by a narrowed portion (or neck)
Line	Similar to a crest but not raised as much (is often rather faint)
Margin	Edge of a flat bone or flat portion of the edge of a flat area
Meatus	Tubelike opening or channel (*pl.*, meatus or meatuses)
Neck	A narrowed portion, usually at the base of a head
Notch	A V-like depression in the margin or edge of a flat area
Process	A raised area or projection
Ramus	Curved portion of a bone, like a ram's horn (*pl.*, rami)
Sinus	Cavity within a bone
Sulcus	Groove or elongated depression (*pl.*, sulci)
Trochanter	Large bump for muscle attachment (larger than tubercle or tuberosity)
Tuberosity	Oblong, raised bump, usually for muscle attachment; also called a *tuber*; a small tuberosity is called a *tubercle*

Table 6.1

Part B: Properties of Bone

Introduction

Bone health is a growing concern in our aging population; osteoporosis affects 1 in 3 women and 1 in 5 men over the age of 50. As health organizations have sought to educate people about bone health, the emphasis has been on how to have strong bones. Studies show that muscle-building activities puts pressure on bones, promoting their growth and increasing bone mineral density. This is especially true for activities that have high impact forces. So perhaps comic book purists can make a scientifically sound claim: The bones of superheroes are stronger than the average human because long years of rigorous training increases their bone mineral density immensely. But bone strength is not the entire picture. Bone flexibility is just as important so that bones can withstand strain without breaking. Bone strength is determined by the matrix, within which bone cells are embedded. The matrix is a framework of inorganic minerals such as calcium. Bone flexibility is conferred by collagenous fibers embedded in the extracellular matrix, (also called *ground substance*). Many of the actions of the body are possible because bones can withstand three different forces: torsional (twisting), compressional (squeezing), and tensile (stretching) forces. These forces are endured because the composition of bone is a blend of small crystalline minerals and thin fibrous hairs of collagen, which are interwoven together.

I. The Effect of Acid on Bone (may also be a demonstration)

Materials

Dilute acetic acid (vinegar), hydrochloric acid, or nitric acid
Beaker
Chicken leg bones
Gloves
Protractor

Before You Begin:

- Be sure to wear gloves when handling the chicken leg bones throughout the experiments.

Procedure

1. Examine the properties of the bone, particularly its flexibility.
2. Pour dilute acid into a beaker and place three chicken bones into the solution. The bones will have to soak in the acid for at least a few days for the calcified portions of the bones to dissolve.
3. Remove the bones from the solution and dry them off. Examine the exterior and interior of the bones. Compare the decalcified bones to the fresh chicken bone and note any physical differences.
4. Using a protractor, test the strength of each bone by bending it at a 5-degree angle for 15 seconds. Repeat the strength test and increase the angle 5 degrees each attempt until the bone breaks. Test all three bones. Using the table provided in your lab report, indicate the angle that the bone broke and the location along the bone where breakage occurred.

II. The Effect of Heat on Bone (may also be a demonstration)

Materials

Oven
Balance
Paper towels
Chicken leg bones
Gloves

Procedure

1. Measure the mass of three uncooked chicken leg bones.
2. Place the bones on a pan and place in an oven preheated at 250° F for 30-45 minutes, or until dry.
3. Remove the bones from the oven and allow them to cool for 10 minutes. Record their mass and compare to the mass before they were cooked. The difference in mass is approximately equal to the mass of the water in the bone, which can be converted into a percentage.
4. Place the chicken bones back into the oven for an additional 1.5 hours, which will cook or destroy the organic portions of the bone.
5. Remove the bones from the oven and allow them to cool for 10 minutes. Examine the exterior and interior of the bones. Compare the heated bones to the normal chicken bone and note the physical differences.
6. Using a protractor, test the strength of each bone by bending it at a 5-degree angle for 15 seconds. Repeat the strength test and increase the angle 5 degrees each attempt until the bone breaks. Test at least three bones. Using the table provided in your lab report, indicate the angle that the bone broke and the location along the bone where breakage occurred.

III. Determining the Age of Bones (may also be a demonstration)

> **Materials**
>
> Microscope
> Prepared slides of compact bone

Procedure

1. As a person gets older, his or her bones change, so an increase in the number of osteons can be observed. Additionally, both the general size of the osteons and diameter of the Haversian canals will be smaller.
2. Select three prepared slides of compact bone.
3. Observe the slides with low-power (40x), then medium-power (100X), and finally with high-power magnification (400X). Use the diaphragm and adjust the light for best viewing.
4. To determine the age of a bone sample, count the total number of osteons visible in the medium power field of view. If the bone sample is large and fills your medium power of view, carefully and accurately count the total number of osteons you see in this field of view. Do not move the bone specimen when counting. Ignore partial osteons without a Haversian canal. Record the number of osteons counted in your lab report.

5. If the bone specimen is smaller and does not completely fill your medium-power field of view, you will have to make osteon counts using high power. Then you will have to calculate the number of osteons that would fill the medium-power field of view.
   a. Determine how many osteons are visible in this high-power field of view by counting the number of Haversian canals. Some may appear black, and others may appear clear. If a canal is only half-visible because it is around the edge of your field of view, you should count it as a 0.5 osteon. Record your count in your lab report.
   b. Randomly move your slide to a new location and repeat your osteon count.
   c. Repeat the above steps to count a total of 10 locations on your bone specimen. Record all counts in your lab report.
   d. Calculate the average number of osteons you counted in the high-power field of view (add up all the osteons you counted and divide by 10). Record your average osteon count with high power in your lab report (round to 2 decimal places).
   e. Use the following formula to calculate how many osteons in this bone specimen would be counted in one medium-power field of view. Record your answer in your lab report (round your answer to the nearest whole number).

$$\begin{array}{l} \text{Total \# osteons counted in one} \\ \text{medium-power field of view} \end{array} = \begin{array}{l} \text{Average \# osteons counted in} \\ \text{one high-power field of view} \end{array} \times 16$$

6. Calculate the age of the bone specimen (based on your osteon counts) by using the following formula. Round your specimen's age to the nearest year.

$$\begin{array}{l} \text{Age of bone} \\ + \\ \text{3 years} \end{array} = \begin{array}{l} \text{Total number of osteons counted} \\ \text{in the entire medium-power field} \\ \text{of view} \end{array} + 8.3 =$$

7. Repeat all measurements and calculations for all three slides. Record all data in your lab report.

Lab Report for 6.2

Section A. Activities for Structure of a Long Bone

1. Identify the internal and external features of a long bone in Figure 6.2:

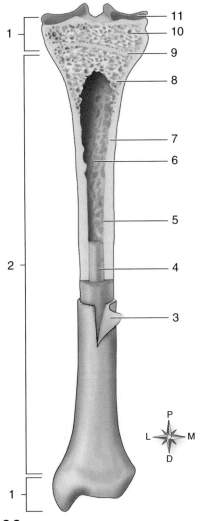

Relevant Terms
_____ Articular cartilage
_____ Compact bone
_____ Diaphysis
_____ Endosteum
_____ Epiphyseal line
_____ Epiphysis
_____ Medullary cavity
_____ Periosteum
_____ Red marrow cavities
_____ Spongy bone
_____ Yellow marrow

Figure 6.2

2. Draw your observations from prepared slides of bone tissue here:

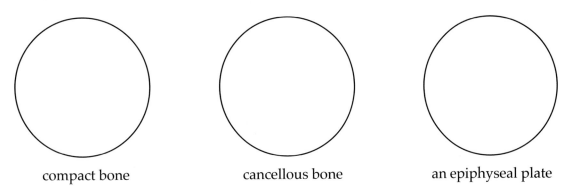

compact bone   cancellous bone   an epiphyseal plate

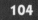

Section B. Activities for Properties of Bone

Description of the fresh chicken bone:

The Effect of Acid on Bone

Description of the decalcified chicken bone:

	Angle						
Trial #1							
Trial #2							
Trial #3							

The Effect of Heat on Bone

Description of the heated chicken bone:
Mass of uncooked chicken bone:

	Mass	Angle						
Trial #1								
Trial #2								
Trial #3								

Determining the Age of Bones

	Bone Specimen 1	Bone Specimen 2	Bone Specimen 3
(If needed) 10 high-power osteon counts and average number of osteons counted with high power			
Total # of osteons counted in an entire medium-power field of view			
Calculated age of bone specimen			

Section C. Assessments

1. T/F   Bones do not produce blood cells.
2. T/F   The ends of long bones are called *epiphyses*.
3. In a long bone, the hollow shaft is called the:
   a. endosteum.
   b. diaphysis.
   c. epiphyses.
   d. periosteum.
4. Cells responsible for bone formation are:
   a. osteons.
   b. osteocytes.
   c. osteoblasts.
   d. chondrocytes.

Section D. Critical Thinking Problems

1. A 2010 article in *Materials Today* asked a simple question, "Why are your bones not made of steel?" Within the article, bioengineering Professor David Taylor explains that steel alloys exist that are ten times better than bone in three important structural properties related to materials engineering: tensile strength, strain to failure, and fracture toughness. He proposes a hypothetical offer: undergo a hospital procedure to have all of the bones in your body replaced with artificial materials.

   What problems might emerge if you were to undergo this procedure?

2. Illegal in major league baseball, a corked baseball bat has had its central wooden portion removed and replaced with a lighter material, such as cork or Styrofoam. Because a corked bat has less mass, the bat can be swung faster but hits the baseball with less efficiency, resulting in a ball that travels at lower speeds and slightly less distance than when hit with a regular bat. Owing to the presumed success of the guise, only six instances have occurred when a baseball player was caught using a corked bat in league play.

   In what way is a bone similar to a corked bat? What advantages and disadvantages does this provide as opposed to a bone that consisted only of compact bone?

Activity #2 — The Axial Skeleton

Part A: The Skull

Introduction

Although Hamlet was able to recall facial features of Yorick, a deceased king's jester from his youth, he initially could not recognize him from his skull alone. The skull is a fundamental component for facial recognition, especially certain surface features of the skull, such as the shape of the orbit and cheekbones. Research into facial recognition suggests that the process by which we perceive others is by viewing the face as a whole rather than a collection of parts, while noting specific features that stand out. This would explain the challenge for investigators to create facial composites of suspects based on eyewitness accounts, as their bottom-up approach to facial reconstruction can overlook global features of the skull.

When it comes to superheroes, much is conveyed about their character in the shape of their skulls. Beyond the handful of comic book characters that lack skin, such as the Ghost Rider, the square jaw lines of Superman and Batman and the Amazonian facial contours of Wonder Woman are iconic, so much so that they have redefined the masculine and feminine ideals the public desires in movie stars.

For all its value in our concept of beauty, the skull interacts with almost all of the organ systems in the body (except for the urinary and reproductive systems). It also houses the brain and multiple sensory systems in addition to serving as the portal for our bodies to acquire food.

> **Materials**
>
> Textbook
> Intact skull
> Beauchene skull
> Articulated human skeleton, for reference

Procedure

1. Review content in your textbook related to the skull.
2. Utilize both the intact and Beauchene skulls to identify markings, cranial bones, and important features of the skull in Figure 6.3.

Part B: Vertebral Column and Thoracic Cage

Introduction

Whether a superhero or an average human, the vertebral column, or spine, is the central anatomical feature of support in the body. The skull rests on it, the thoracic cage emerges from it and the lower and upper extremities attach to it. Furthermore, it houses the pipeline of communication from the brain to the rest of the body: the spinal cord. Because all the other organ systems are contained by or connect to the skeletal system through muscular or connective tissue, the spine carries the weight of the body. However, unlike man-made structures built for support, which tend to be rigid or made from tough materials, the vertebral column is segmented, permitting flexibility in lateral directions, and has intercalated, cartilaginous discs between vertebrae, allowing for vertical compressions.

Just as the skull protects the brain, the thoracic cage or bony thorax similarly protects the heart and lungs as well as other vital organs. However, unlike the hard, fused bones of the skull, the organs within the torso are protected by stacked, arc-shaped ribs intercalated with intercostal muscles. The ribs stem from the vertebrae and curve inward to connect to the long, flat sternum, collectively creating an overall egg shape.

Materials

Articulated human skeleton
Disarticulated human skeleton

Procedure

1. Review content in your textbook related to the vertebral column and thoracic cage.
2. Using the models of the skeleton as a guide, identify the vertebrae in Figure 6.4 and Figure 6.5
3. Using the models of the skeleton as a guide, identify the thoracic cage in Figure 6.6.

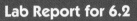

Lab Report for 6.2

Section A. Activities for the Skull

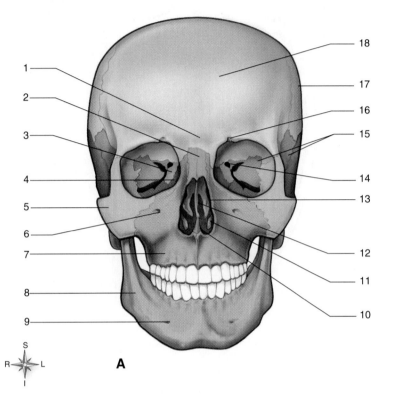

Figure 6.3

Figure 6.3 (con't)

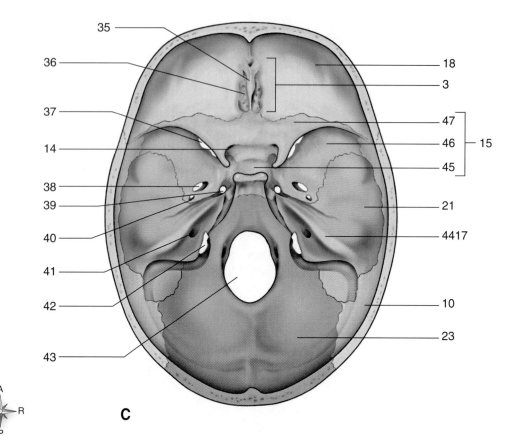

C

Figure 6.3 (con't)

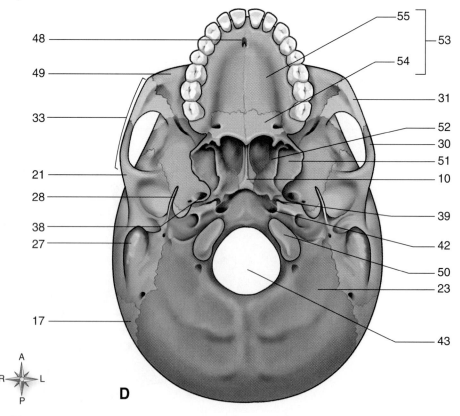

D

Figure 6.3 (con't)

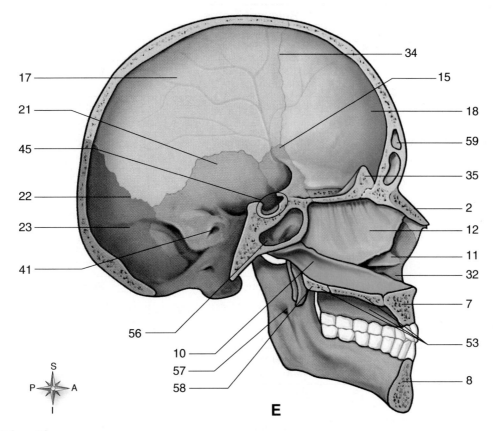

Figure 6.3 (con't)

Relevant Terms		
Cranial Bones	_____ External acoustic meatus	_____ Medial pterygoid plate of sphenoid
_____ Ethmoid bone	_____ External occipital protuberance	_____ Mental foramen of mandible
_____ Frontal bone	_____ Foramen lacerum	_____ Middle nasal concha of ethmoid bone
_____ Inferior nasal concha	_____ Foramen magnum	_____ Occipital condyle
_____ Lacrimal bone	_____ Foramen ovale	_____ Optic foramen of sphenoid bone
_____ Mandible	_____ Foramen spinosum	_____ Palatine process of maxilla
_____ Maxilla	_____ Frontal process of maxilla	_____ Perpendicular plate of ethmoid bone
_____ Nasal bone	_____ Frontal sinus	_____ Petrous part of temporal bone
_____ Occipital bone	_____ Glabella	_____ Pterygoid process of sphenoid bone
_____ Palatine bone	_____ Greater wing of sphenoid bone	_____ Sella turcica of sphenoid bone
_____ Parietal bone	_____ Hard palate	_____ Sphenoid air sinus
_____ Sphenoid bone	_____ Incisive foramen of maxilla	_____ Squamous suture
_____ Temporal bone	_____ Infraorbital foramen of maxilla	_____ Styloid process
_____ Vomer	_____ Internal acoustic meatus	_____ Superior and inferior temporal lines
_____ Zygomatic bone	_____ Jugular foramen	_____ Superior orbital fissure
Cranial Features and Markings	_____ Lambdoid suture	_____ Supraorbital foramen of frontal bone
_____ Condyloid process of mandible	_____ Lateral pterygoid plate of sphenoid	_____ Temporal process of zygomatic bone
_____ Coronal suture	_____ Lesser wing of sphenoid bone	_____ Zygomatic arch
_____ Cribriform plate	_____ Mandibular foramen	_____ Zygomatic process of maxilla
_____ Crista galli of ethmoid bone	_____ Mastoid process of temporal bone	_____ Zygomatic process of temporal bone

Section B. Activities for Vertebral Column and Thoracic Cage

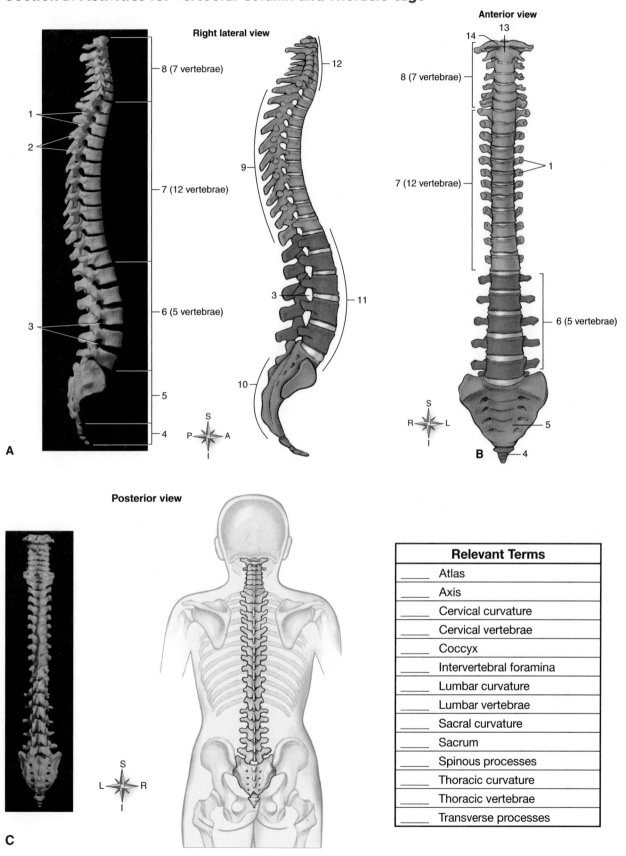

Right lateral view

8 (7 vertebrae)

1

2

7 (12 vertebrae)

6 (5 vertebrae)

3

5

4

A

12

9

3

11

10

Anterior view

14

13

8 (7 vertebrae)

1

7 (12 vertebrae)

6 (5 vertebrae)

5

4

B

Posterior view

C

Figure 6.4

Relevant Terms
_____ Atlas
_____ Axis
_____ Cervical curvature
_____ Cervical vertebrae
_____ Coccyx
_____ Intervertebral foramina
_____ Lumbar curvature
_____ Lumbar vertebrae
_____ Sacral curvature
_____ Sacrum
_____ Spinous processes
_____ Thoracic curvature
_____ Thoracic vertebrae
_____ Transverse processes

Atlas, superior view

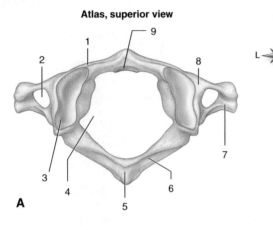

A

Atlas, lateral view

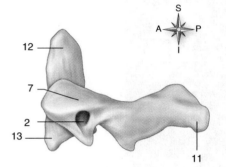

Axis, superior view

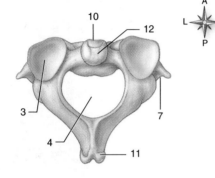

B

Axis, lateral view

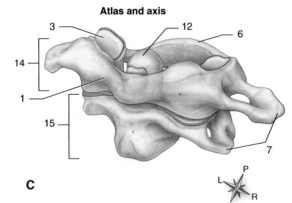

Atlas and axis

C

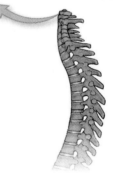

Figure 6.5

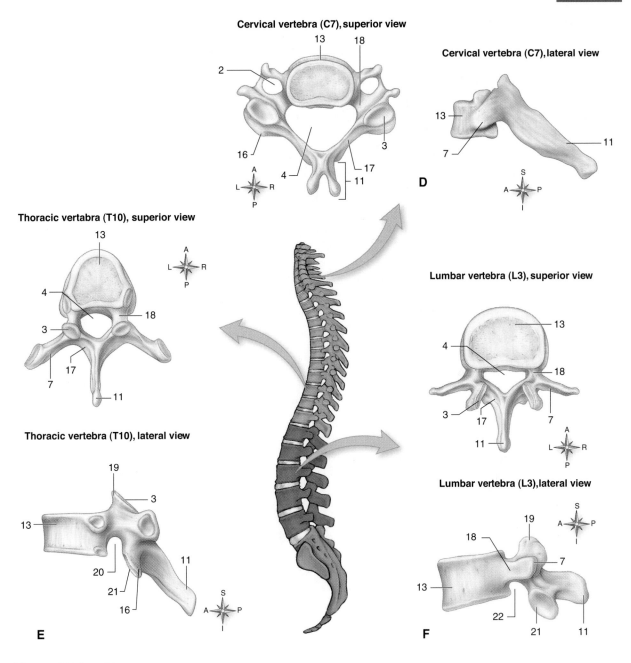

Cervical vertebra (C7), superior view

Cervical vertebra (C7), lateral view

D

Thoracic vertabra (T10), superior view

Lumbar vertebra (L3), superior view

Thoracic vertebra (T10), lateral view

Lumbar vertebra (L3), lateral view

E

F

Figure 6.5 (con't)

Relevant Terms		
_____ Anterior arch	_____ Inferior articular process	_____ Spinous process
_____ Anterior articular facet	_____ Inferior vertebral notch	_____ Superior articular facet
_____ Atlas	_____ Lamina	_____ Superior articular process
_____ Axis	_____ Lateral mass	_____ Superior vertebral notch
_____ Body	_____ Pedicle	_____ Transverse foramen
_____ Dens	_____ Posterior arch	_____ Transverse process
_____ Facet (for dens of axis)	_____ Posterior tubercle	_____ Vertebral foramen
_____ Inferior articular facet		

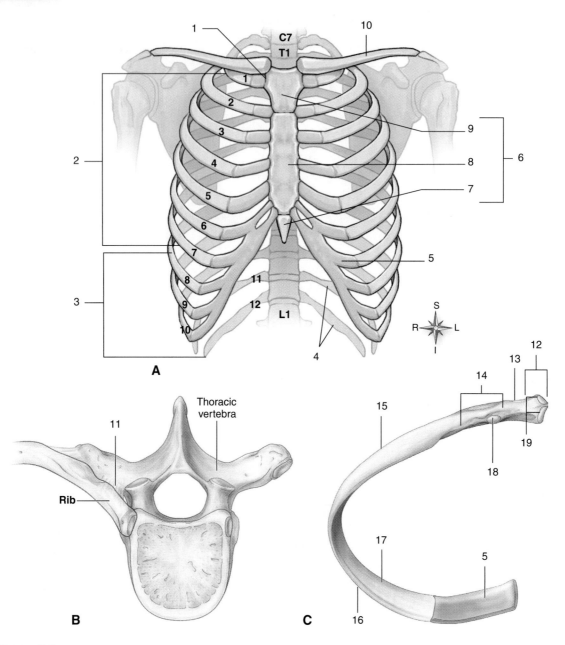

Figure 6.6

Relevant Terms		
_____ Articular facet (for transverse process of vertebra)	_____ Costosternal articulation	_____ Ligaments
_____ Articular facets (for ventral body)	_____ External surface	_____ Manubrium
_____ Body	_____ False ribs	_____ Neck
_____ Clavicle	_____ Floating ribs	_____ Sternum
_____ Costal cartilage	_____ Head	_____ True ribs
_____ Costal groove	_____ Internal surface	_____ Xiphoid process
_____ Costal tubercle		

Section C. Assessments

1. T/F The occipital bone is located at the back of the skull.
2. T/F In order from superior to inferior, the sequence of the vertebrae is cervical, thoracic, lumbar, coccyx, and sacrum.
3. T/F The curves of the spine help to support the body's weight.
4. T/F The palatine bone is the cheekbone.
5. The upper jaw bone is called the:
   a. zygomatic.
   b. ethmoid bone.
   c. maxilla.
   d. mandible.
6. Which of the following bones is NOT in the skull?
   a. parietal bone
   b. xiphoid process
   c. temporal bone
   d. vomer
7. Ribs that do not attach to costal cartilage at all are:
   a. true ribs.
   b. false ribs.
   c. floating ribs.
   d. All ribs attach to costal cartilage.
8. Which section of the vertebral column contains the most vertebrae?
   a. cervical section
   b. thoracic section
   c. lumbar section
   d. sacrum section

Section D. Critical Thinking Problems

1. From birth, the development of the skull occurs through the growth, ossification and fusion of hundreds of fibrous and cartilage structures. What problems might occur if this process began much earlier during *in utero* development?

2. Even though both protect vital organs, what advantage is there for both humans and animals in a rib cage that lacks fused bones, such as those of the skull?

3. Snakes have hundreds of vertebrae, which accounts for their unique locomotion. Why would hundreds of vertebrae in humans be problematic?

4. In which planes does the spine move? How do our spinal movements compare to those of a fish? A whale? Does this reflect evolutionary connections to other mammals?

Activity #3 — The Appendicular Skeleton

Part A: Pectoral Girdle and Upper Extremity

Introduction

We may not often think about how our upper limbs are attached to our bodies, but it's quite a marvel, considering that only two bones are involved. The pectoral girdle rests on top of the thoracic cage, with the clavicle arching between the sternum and acromion of the scapula in the front while the rest of the scapula hugs around the backside of the ribs. The glenoid cavity is notched in such a way that the head of the humerus fits within it, allowing for a large degree of motion. Action movies often depict getting shot in the shoulder as a "minor" wound, when in fact it is quite serious with the potential of permanent complications.

At the other end of the upper extremity, the 27 bones in each hand are organized and splayed out to allow for all the tasks required of them, whether working independently or cooperatively. With the flexibility provided by the joint at the elbow, the bones of the upper extremity allow for all the action-packed movements of both humans and superheroes alike.

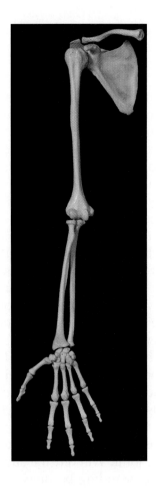

Materials

Textbook
Articulated human skeleton
Disarticulated human skeleton

Procedure

1. Review content in your textbook related to the pectoral girdle and upper extremity.
2. Refer to both skeleton models in order to identify the features in Figure 6.8.

Part B: Pelvic Girdle and Lower Extremity

Introduction

Unlike the pectoral girdle that creates a lateral extension for upper-limb attachment, the pelvic girdle functions as a support for the torso, which makes contact with the sacrum of the vertebral column at the point of ilium of each pelvic coxal bone. Functionally, the weight of the body rests on the pelvic girdle, which redistributes force into the lower extremities. The ring of the pelvis is completed as the pubic crest of each bone sandwiches a cartilaginous joint called the *pubic symphysis*, forming the pubic arch. Though this simple structural approach provides an incredible amount of support for the upper portion of the body, it is not without its weaknesses.

For all the punches to the body and face that superheroes use to thrash their villains, a simple lesson from self-defense experts could make the fight end faster. As shown in the TV show *Fight Science*, a basic but forceful strike to the pelvic region can fracture the pelvic girdle at the pubic joint. Without the support of the pelvic girdle, standing becomes difficult and walking is impossible. Perhaps superheroes do not utilize this move because they are respecting boxing rules by not hitting "below the belt."

The lower extremities follow a similar structural pattern as the upper extremities but are functionally different in that the lower extremities are the sole support of the bipedal human. Ultimately, the force of the body weight is distributed between just two bones of each foot: the talus and calcaneus, which are tarsal bones in the posterior portion of the foot and form part of the ankle. Not surprisingly, self-defense experts also target this area to immobilize someone posing a threat.

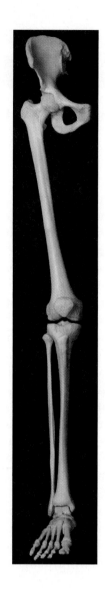

Materials

Textbook
Articulated human skeleton
Disarticulated human skeleton

Procedure

1. Review content in your textbook related to the pelvic girdle and lower extremity.
2. Identify the bones of the lower extremities in Figure 6.10.

Lab Report for 6.3

Section A. Activities for the Pectoral Girdle and Upper Extremity

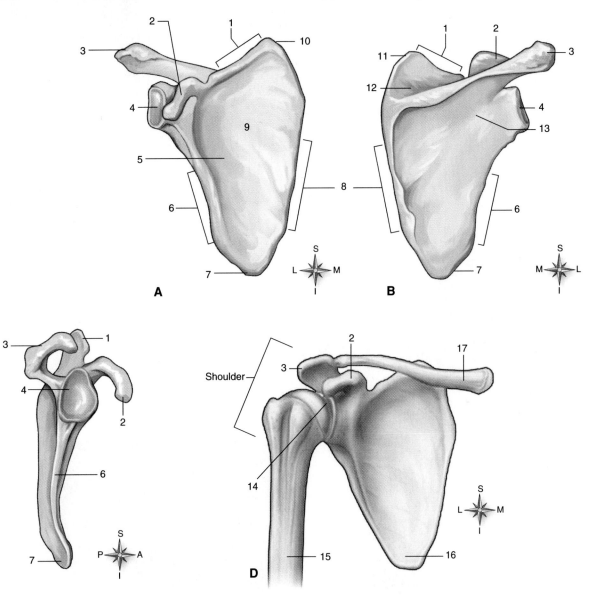

Figure 6.8

Relevant Terms		
_____ Acromion	_____ Humerus	_____ Scapula
_____ Clavicle	_____ Inferior angle	_____ Subscapular fossa
_____ Coracoid process	_____ Infraspinous fossa	_____ Superior angle
_____ Costal surface	_____ Lateral (axillary) border	_____ Superior border
_____ Glenohumoral joint	_____ Medial (vertebral) border	_____ Supraspinous fossa
_____ Glenoid cavity	_____ Medial angle	

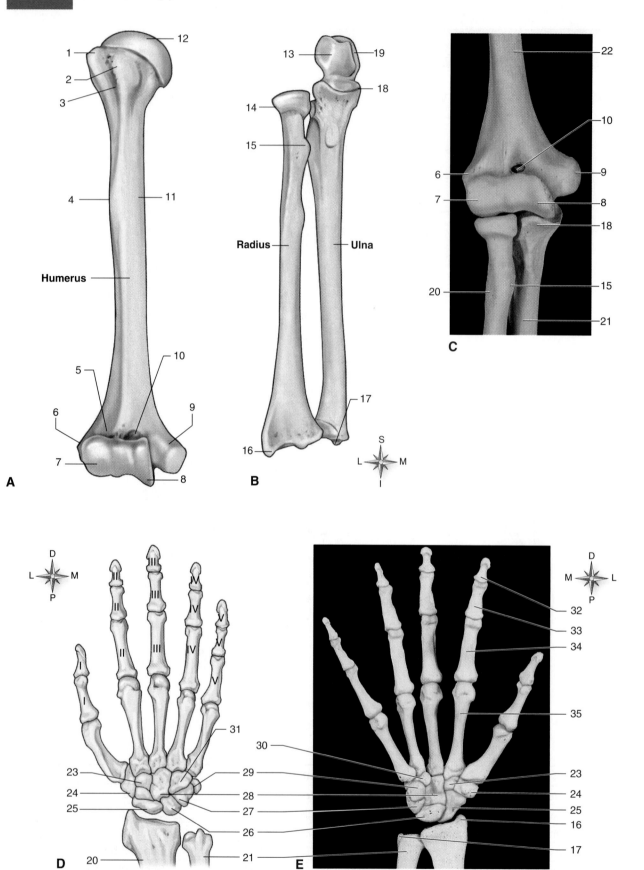

A

B

C

D

E

Radius

Ulna

Humerus

Figure 6.8 (con't)

Relevant Terms		
_____ Capitate	_____ Intertubercular groove	_____ Radial tuberosity
_____ Capitulum	_____ Lateral epicondyle	_____ Radius
_____ Coronoid fossa	_____ Lesser tubercle	_____ Scaphoid
_____ Coronoid process	_____ Lunate	_____ Styloid process of radius
_____ Deltoid tuberosity	_____ Medial epicondyle	_____ Styloid process of ulna
_____ Distal phalanx	_____ Metacarpal bone	_____ Trapezium
_____ Greater tubercle	_____ Middle phalanx	_____ Trapezoid
_____ Hamate	_____ Nutrient foramen	_____ Triquetrum
_____ Hamate hook	_____ Olecranon process	_____ Trochlea
_____ Head	_____ Pisiform	_____ Trochlear notch
_____ Head of radius	_____ Proximal phalanx	_____ Ulna
_____ Humerus	_____ Radial fossa	

Section B. Activities for the Pelvic Girdle and Lower Extremity

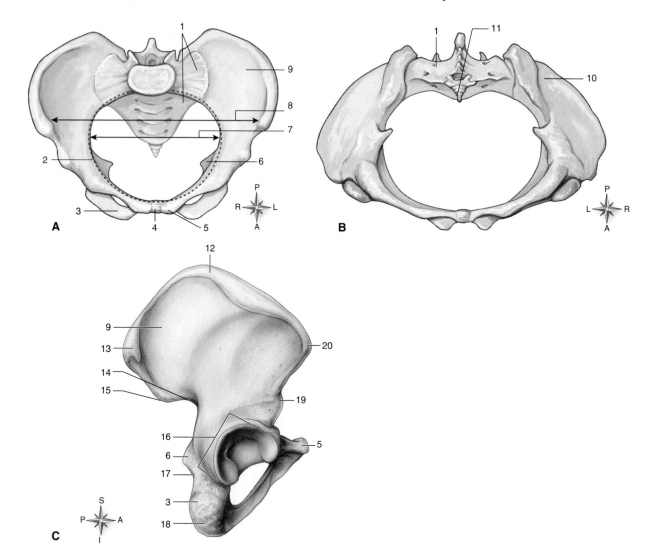

Figure 6.10

Relevant Terms		
_____ Adductor tubercle	_____ Intercondylar fossa	_____ Middle phalanx
_____ Calcaneus	_____ Lateral condyle	_____ Navicular bones
_____ Crest	_____ Lateral epicondyle	_____ Neck of femur
_____ Cuboid bone	_____ Lateral malleolus	_____ Patella
_____ Cuneiform bones	_____ Lesser trochanter	_____ Patellar surface
_____ Distal phalanx	_____ Linea aspera	_____ Phalanges
_____ Femur	_____ Medial condyle	_____ Proximal phalanx
_____ Fibula	_____ Medial epicondyle	_____ Talus
_____ Greater trochanter	_____ Medial malleolus	_____ Tibia
_____ Head of femur	_____ Medial supracondylar line	_____ Tibial tuberosity
_____ Head of fibula	_____ Metatarsal bones	

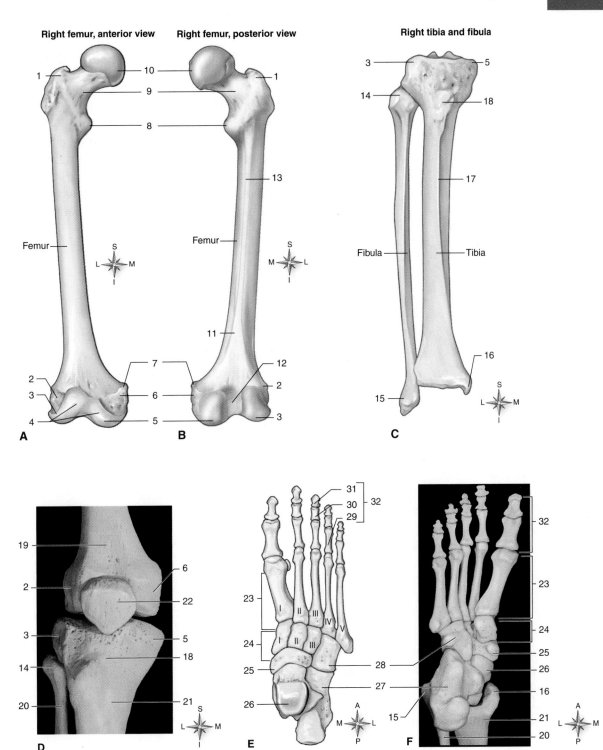

Figure 6.10 (con't)

Section C. Assessments

1. T/F   The male and female skeletons differ in the shape of the pelvis.
2. T/F   The patella is above the kneecap.
3. T/F   The olecranon process is another term for the elbow.
4. The bones of the lower arm are the:
   a. tibia and fibula.
   b. ulna and radius.
   c. femur and humerus.
   d. clavicle and scapula.
5. The tarsals are located in the:
   a. wrist.
   b. hand.
   c. foot.
   d. ankle.
6. There are ____ phalanges in the body.
   a. 14
   b. 28
   c. 56
   d. 84

Section D. Critical Thinking Problems

1. A common injury to an infant during birth is a broken clavicle. How might this occur?

2. In humans, both the bones of the forearm and leg are bifurcated. This is not the case in horses. When is bifurcation more structurally advantageous than a single bone? Would two bones be better at the arm and thigh?

3. In 2009, a boy was born in the San Francisco area with a fully functioning set of 12 fingers and 12 toes. His condition, known as *polydactylism*, is not new. Many people born with an extra finger or toe have them surgically removed after birth because they are often nonfunctioning or parents opt to protect their children from the social stigma. What advantage might this boy have over other children that would take him a step closer to being a superhero?

4. During fetal ultrasound, two measurements that are commonly taken are the humerus and femur lengths at specific weeks of gestation. Considering the variation in human height, what value is there in taking these measurements?

Activity #4 — Joints

Introduction

When developing a machine, engineers must find ways to minimize the heat generated by moving parts and avoid having them come into direct contact with each other, which would create friction. This friction can be incredibly detrimental to a machine when it is not lubricated with a substance that allows for fluid motion, such as might happen to a car engine that lacks motor oil.

The skeletal system also has moving parts that are close to one another. The junctions that bones form are called *joints* or *articulations* and it is here that the issue of friction is handled beautifully by the human body through the use synovial fluid. Furthermore, just as machined parts are contoured to one another, the shapes and surface features of bone around joints permit movement and complement each other.

Materials

Textbook
Articulated human skeleton
Disarticulated human skeleton
Model of various joints

Procedure

1. Review content in your textbook related to joints.
2. Classify the various joints in Figure 6.11 by their type.
3. Refer to both skeleton models in order to identify the joints in Figure 6.12.
4. For each joint in the body, be sure you are able to identify the type of joint it represents and the kind of motion it permits.

Lab Report for 6.4

Section A. Activities

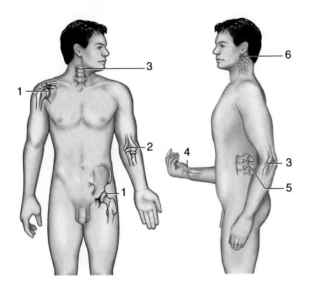

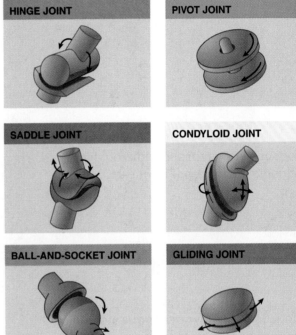

Figure 6.11

Relevant Terms
_____ Ball and socket joint
_____ Condyloid joint
_____ Gliding joint
_____ Hinge joint
_____ Pivot joint
_____ Saddle joint

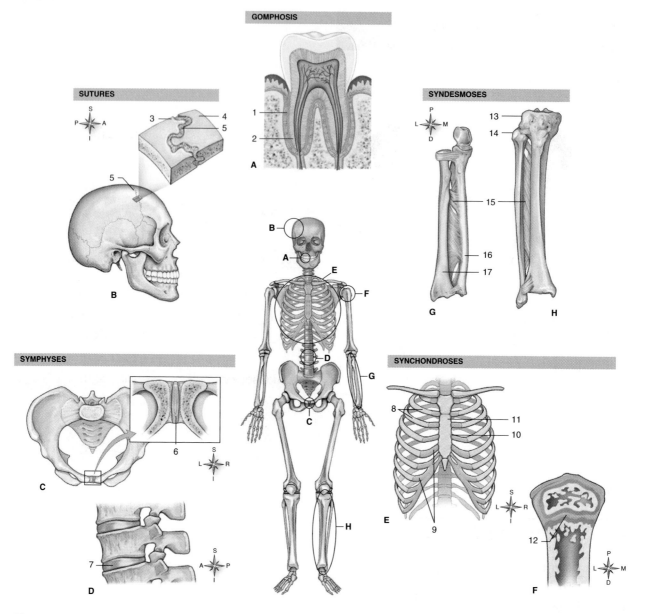

Figure 6.12

Relevant Terms		
_____ Costal cartilage	_____ Parietal bone	_____ Sternum
_____ Costosternal synchondrosis	_____ Periodontal membrane (made of periodontal ligaments)	_____ Suture
_____ Epiphyseal plate (hyaline cartilage)	_____ Pubic symphysis	_____ Tibia
_____ Fibula	_____ Radius	_____ Ulna
_____ Frontal bone	_____ Ribs	_____ Vertebral disk
_____ Interosseus ligament	_____ Root of tooth in socket	

Section B. Assessments

1. T/F   A joint that cannot move is a fibrous joint.
2. T/F   The hip is a cartilaginous joint.
3. Match the following joint types with their representative examples.

ball and socket	___	Between the proximal phalanges and metacarpal bones
condyloid	___	Head of the radius against the radial notch of ulna
gliding	___	Between the carpal and tarsal bones
hinge	___	Knee
pivot	___	Shoulder
saddle	___	Between the radius and carpal bones

Section C. Critical Thinking Problems

1. Viscosity is the measure of a fluid's resistance to flow. An interesting property of the synovial fluid in a synovial joint is that its viscosity is not constant. In fact, its viscosity decreases the longer the joint is moved. In what ways is this a beneficial property of synovial fluid? What if the opposite were true?

2. Lana Lang, Superman's romantic interest from Smallville, once rescued an insect-like alien who nearly died. In thanks, the alien gave Lana a ring that allowed her to have the powers of arthropods by morphing the lower half of her body into any insect or arachnid on a daily basis, allowing Lana to become the Insect Queen.

   Arthropods have jointed legs, which have hinges where the hard exoskeleton is softer at the joint. This means that various portions of the exoskeleton come into contact with each other. Would this actually be better than regular human joints?

Exercise 7
The Muscular System

Lesson Overview

Activity #1: Muscle Structure and Function
    Part A: Single Muscle Fiber Contraction
    Part B: In-Vivo Contraction of Human Muscle Tissue
Activity #2: Muscles of the Head and Face
Activity #3: Muscles of the Core
Activity #4: Muscles of the Upper and Lower Extremities

Overview

Consider two healthy men, equal in all aspects, including physique, diet, and genetics, except that one can do multiple biceps curls with a 40-pound weight while the other can handle 70 pounds with ease. Whether the second man is healthier than the first is difficult to say. The major difference between the two lies in the muscles of their upper extremities. On a day-to-day basis, the ability to utilize these muscles to lift 5-10 pounds is sufficient for their basic survival. Unlike superheroes, whose excep-tional strength is called upon day after day to save people, it's unlikely that the ability to lift a 50-pound object is a life or death matter in the lives of these men.

To begin the study of the muscular system, we examine the structure of muscle itself, and then continue much in the same way as we did with the skeletal system, beginning with the muscles of the head and face, then the torso, and finally the upper and lower extremities.

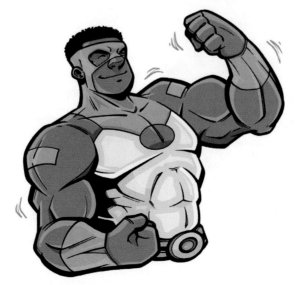

Activity #1 — Muscle Structure and Function

Part A: Single Muscle Fiber Contraction

Introduction

In the comic book world, superheroes do not always opt to work alone, as Batman notoriously preferred. The Justice League and the Avengers are teams of superheroes that join forces to stand up against villains greater than any one of them could face alone. The stories of their adventures serve as lessons in cooperation and what can be accomplished when peo-ple work together, combining their strengths to maximize their effectiveness.

An even better example of cooperation can be found in skeletal muscles. The structure of skeletal muscle can be thought of as cords within cords within cords, all working together to produce the voluntary motions we can achieve with our bodies.

To investigate muscle characteristics in depth, we need to scale down to the level of the individual fiber itself to unravel the molecular basis of muscle function. Although direct observation of sarcomere contraction is a challenge, in this lab it is possible to observe the contraction of a single muscle fiber using an appropriate kit.

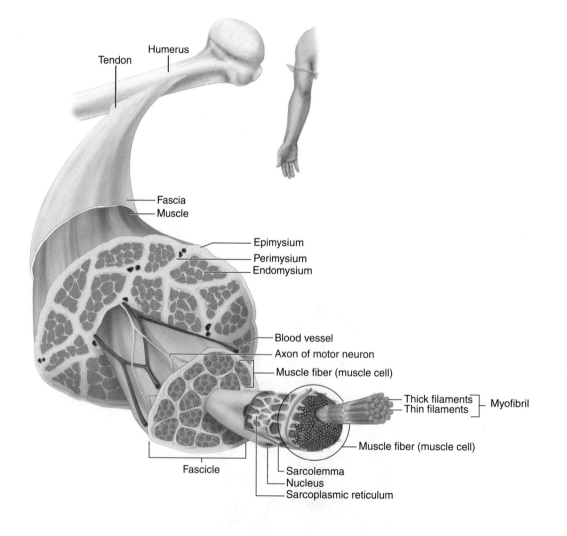

Part B: In-Vivo Contraction of Human Muscle Tissue

Materials

Glycerinated skeletal muscle tissue
Pipettes or medicine droppers
Teasing needles
Millimeter ruler
Forceps
Petri dishes
Microscope, slides, and coverslips

Before You Begin

- *You will conduct the following activity as a team. It is important that you are organized and delegate tasks appropriately to ensure that the experiment is a success and materials are not wasted.*
- *If a kit is used for this activity, it may be worthwhile to review the included instructions on how to use the materials.*
- *It is important that the kit materials are frozen and/or refrigerated, when appropriate.*

Procedure

1. Review the section in your textbook referring to muscle tissue.
2. Familiarize yourself with the muscle kit, the materials, and the instructions provided.
3. Be sure to acquire thinner strands, as thicker muscle fibers (thicker than a few tenths of a millimeter) may not contract.
4. Examine muscle fibers with the microscope. Measure the length of a few muscle fibers before and after applying an ATP solution in order to calculate the change in length of the fiber as a result of contraction. Contraction is fairly rapid but may vary depending on solutions and technique.

Introduction

Villains in comic books typically have two major obsessions: (1) seeking power, fame, or wealth, or (2) incapacitating superheroes, because they typically get in the way of the first obsession. One standard villainous plot is to somehow gain control over a superhero's mind or body and enslave him or her for evil purposes. This is usually followed by a long-winded monologue peppered with maniacal laughter as the superhero is forced to do the master's bidding.

Many of the organs in the human body function involuntarily, with the skeletal muscles being an obvious exception. Muscles that twitch or begin to spasm can be annoying, in part because they are beyond our control. But muscles in your body can be stimulated electrically from a source other than your own nervous system, which can be quite displacing — providing a small sense of what superheroes endure at the hands of their archenemies.

Materials

Textbook
Physiogrip, PowerLab, or alternative apparatus for *in-vivo* muscle contraction
Procedures and instruction for proper use of this equipment

Before You Begin

- *Do NOT participate in this activity if you have any health problems sensitive to electrical impulses, such as a heart condition (pacemakers). Keep in mind that the human body can conduct electricity and therefore the subject should not touch anyone or anything other than the appropriate part of the apparatus during the procedure.*

Procedure

1. Review the section in your textbook referring to muscles of the forearm.
2. Identify the components of a muscle in Figure 7.3.
3. Familiarize yourself with the apparatus, the materials, and the instructions.
4. Your instructor will detail the proper use of the apparatus and the procedure to obtain the best results, depending on the apparatus used. The goal is to experience and observe the contraction of muscles in your arm and hand with the minimum voltage possible.

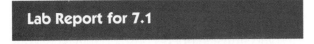

Lab Report for 7.1

Section A. Activities for Single Muscle Fiber Contraction

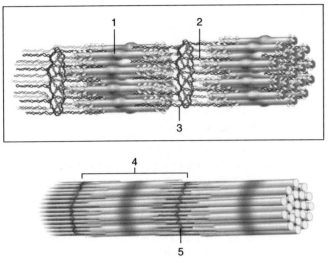

1.
2.
3.
4.
5.

Figure 7.3

Section B. Activities for In-Vivo Contraction of Human Muscle Tissue

Use the following space to record observations related to the Human Muscle Contraction activity as well as any additional information your instructor assigns.

Description of muscle fiber before measurement:_____

_____

_____

_____

Initial length of the muscle fiber(s): _____

Description of muscle fiber before measurement:_____

_____

_____

_____

Final length of the muscle fiber(s): _____

Section C. Assessments

1. T/F Another term for skeletal muscle is *involuntary muscle.*
2. T/F All muscles contract.
3. T/F Actin is the thin myofilament in a muscle fiber.
4. The connective tissue that attaches muscle to bone is:
    a. origin.
    b. bursae.
    c. fascicle.
    d. tendon.
5. The basic contractile unit of a skeletal muscle is the:
    a. sarcomere.
    b. actin.
    c. myosin.
    d. None of the above.
6. Muscle contraction occurs when:
    a. actin shortens
    b. myosin shortens.
    c. the Z-lines are pulled closer together.
    d. both a and b.

Section D. Critical Thinking Problems

1. Once muscle fibers contract, they stay contracted. How do the muscle fibers in the human body get stretched out again?

2. It is possible to keep muscles contracted until fatigue, a process known as *tetanus,* simply by providing many stimuli per second. This also causes the muscle to have a greater contraction than in a single stimulus. If a league of villains were hatching a plan to beat superheroes, how could they use this information to their advantage? What are some of the drawbacks of this approach?

Activity #2 — Muscles of the Head and Face

Introduction

In the 70 years since comic books were first created, one aspect that has changed significantly is the more realistic depictions found in illustrations. With this evolution of comic illustration has also come a shift in the quality of the storytelling. The stories during the Golden Age of comics were driven primarily by narrator blocks and word/thought balloons, but modern comics are able to convey much greater emotional and psychological conflict due to the more sophisticated level of illustration. This evolution has transformed comics into a rich palette of artistic media, including graphic novels, animation, and film.

Even a cursory glance at comic books allows one to sense the feelings of superheroes because so much emotion is captured in their faces. An eyebrow raised, a turned corner of the mouth, or a head drooping down convey much about the inner thoughts of the superhero. The plethora of facial expressions is possible because of the 43 muscles of the face, which are important not only for nonverbal communication, but also speech and mastication. Together, these muscles serve multiple functions in what is often the central focus of the human figure.

Materials

Textbook
Human skull model with musculature, if available

Procedure

1. Review content in your textbook related to the muscles of the head and face.
2. For the purpose of identification and/or for review, demonstrate the contractions of each muscle as you proceed through this lab. Additionally, be sure to locate the origins and insertions of each muscle on your body, where possible, their span, and location relative to other muscles and bones.
3. Refer to the model and to your own or a partner's face to identify the muscles in Figure 7.4.

Lab Report for 7.2

Section A. Activities for Muscles of the Head and Face

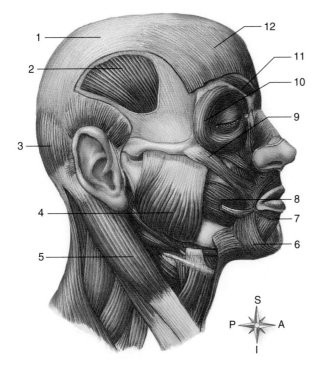

Figure 7.4

Relevant Terms
_____ Buccinator
_____ Corrugator supercilii
_____ Depressor anguli oris
_____ Epicranial aponeurosis
_____ Masseter
_____ Occipitofrontalis
_____ Occipitofrontalis
_____ Orbicularis oculi
_____ Orbicularis oris
_____ Sternocleidomastoid
_____ Temporalis
_____ Zygomaticus major

Section B. Assessments

1. T/F   The sternocleidomastoid moves the neck forward.
2. T/F   Orbicularis oculi is also known as the "kissing" muscle.
3. T/F   The origin of the temporalis is the mandible.
4. Which of the following muscles is NOT a muscle of the head and neck?
    a. buccinator
    b. brachialis
    c. masseter
    d. zygomaticus
5. To close your mouth, which of the following muscles are involved?
    a. masseter
    b. temporalis
    c. orbicularis oris
    d. all of the above
6. The muscle responsible for pulling down the lower lip is the:
    a. platysma.
    b. orbicularis oris.
    c. masseter.
    d. frontalis.

Section C. Critical Thinking Problem

1. Is there anything super about superhero faces? Explain your answer.

Activity #3 — Muscles of the Core

Introduction

Infomercials advertising specialized exercise programs and equipment occasionally suggest that they "target your body's core," but where exactly is your core? Simply put, these are the muscles central to supporting the torso and muscles that keep your head, arms, and legs attached to it. Thus, the core includes the layers of muscles in the neck, thoracic cage, vertebral column, abdominal wall, and pelvis. Depending on how they are classified, muscles of the shoulder and hip, which are important for supporting the attachment of the extremities to the torso, can be considered as part of the core.

Core muscles are important for static support, such as for posture and protection of vital organs, and more dynamic processes that require varying degrees of flexibility, including activities such as breathing and the transfer of force from your legs to your arms, a vital technique in martial arts. Hence, they affect strength, endurance, control, and power, each of which affects the health and physical capabilities of the average human, and even more so, the average superhero. While strengthening the core produces desirable muscular features for regular people, such as washboard abs, the superhero presumably has well-defined core muscles due to laborious training for action. Beyond giving superheroes their shapely masculine and feminine builds, a strong core is essential to fighting well, and for the superhero, it may be the difference between life and death.

Materials

Textbook
Human torso model with musculature, if available

Procedure

1. Review content in your textbook related to the muscles of the core.
2. For the purpose of identification and/or for review, demonstrate the contractions of each muscle as you proceed through this lab. Additionally, be sure to locate the origins and insertions of each muscle on your body, where possible, their span, and location relative to other muscles and bones.
3. Refer to the model and to your own or partner's neck, back, and pelvis to identify the muscles in Figure 7.5a and 7.5b.

Lab Report for 7.3

Section A. Activities for Muscles of the Core

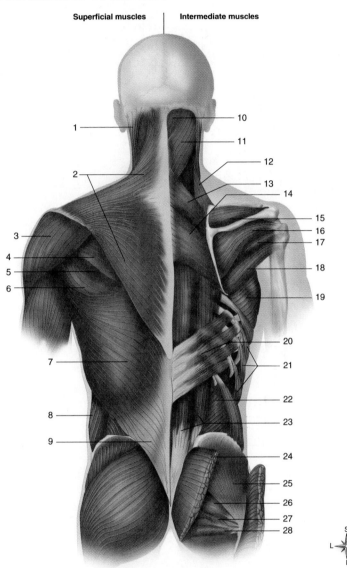

Figure 7.5a

Relevant Terms		
Superficial Muscles	**Intermediate Muscles**	
_____ Deltoid	_____ Erector spinae	_____ Rhomboideus minor
_____ External abdominal oblique	_____ External abdominal oblique	_____ Semispinalis capitis
_____ Infraspinatus	_____ Gluteus maximus	_____ Serratus anterior
_____ Latissimus dorsi	_____ Gluteus medius	_____ Serratus posterior inferior
_____ Sternocleidomastoid	_____ Inferior gemellus	_____ Splenius capitis
_____ Teres major	_____ Infraspinatus	_____ Superior gemellus
_____ Teres minor	_____ Internal abdominal oblique	_____ Supraspinatus
_____ Thoracolumbar fascia	_____ Levator scapulae	_____ Teres major
_____ Trapezius	_____ Piriformis	

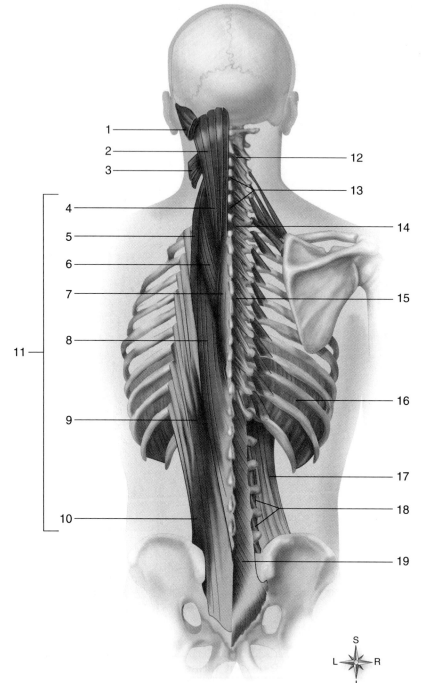

Figure 7.5b

Relevant Terms		
_____ Diaphragm	_____ Levator scapulae	_____ Quadratus lumborum
_____ Erector spinae	_____ Longissimus capitis	_____ Semispinalis capitis
_____ Iliocostalis cervicis	_____ Longissimus cervicis	_____ Semispinalis cervicis
_____ Iliocostalis lumborum	_____ Longissimus thoracis	_____ Semispinalis thoracis
_____ Iliocostalis thoracis	_____ Multifidus (cervical portion)	_____ Spinalis thoracis
_____ Interspinales	_____ Multifidus (lumbar portion)	_____ Splenius capitis
_____ Intertransversarii		

Section B. Assessments

1. T/F   Deep back muscles do little to help with posture.
2. Which of the following is NOT a muscle of the abdominal wall?
   a. rectus abdominis
   b. trapezius
   c. internal oblique
   d. external oblique
3. Match the following muscles to their functions:

Serratus anterior	___	Pulls the shoulder down and forward
Transversus abdominis	___	Rotates the trunk laterally
Diaphragm	___	Enlarges thorax
Semispinalis thoracis	___	Extends the spine
Psoas major	___	Bends the trunk laterally
Internal intercostals	___	Depress the ribs

Section C. Critical Thinking Problems

1. Why would strengthening your core muscles improve balance and posture?

2. Many people suffer from back pain, which can be caused from a variety of issues. How can underdeveloped muscles throughout the core cause pain in the back?

Activity #4 — Muscles of the Upper and Lower Extremities

Materials

Textbook
Muscular models of the upper and lower extremities

Introduction

Combat.

For superheroes, preparing for combat involves instruction in one or many forms of martial arts with intense conditioning. This is essential for success, unless you are The Hulk and can win a battle with a fighting philosophy of "Hulk SMASH!!" Martial arts are ideal for superheroes as the focus is on defensive positions rather than aggressive ones, and proper training ultimately involves figuring how to manipulate arms and legs both for striking and grappling opponents.

Due to the layers of musculature in the upper and lower extremities, the limbs can achieve many positions. People who have developed their arm and leg muscles through training are often lauded and deemed more attractive as large, well-defined biceps and huge quadriceps are viewed as signs of strength. In addition, muscles in the hands and forearms permit an enormous number of manipulations while the 20 muscles in the feet help maintain stance and posture. In this activity, you will see how many of these muscles you can identify in your extremities or a partner's.

Procedure

1. Review content in your textbook related to the muscles of the upper and lower extremities.
2. For the purpose of identification and/or for review, demonstrate the contractions of each muscle as you proceed through this lab. Additionally, be sure to locate the origins and insertions of each muscle on your body, where possible, their span, and location relative to other muscles and bones.
3. Refer to the model and to your own or your partner's arms to identify the muscles of the upper extremities in Figures 7.6a and 7.6b.
4. Refer to the model and to your own or your partner's legs to identify the muscles of the lower extremities in Figures 7.7a and 7.7b.

Lab Report for 7.4

Section A. Activities for Muscles of the Upper and Lower Extremities

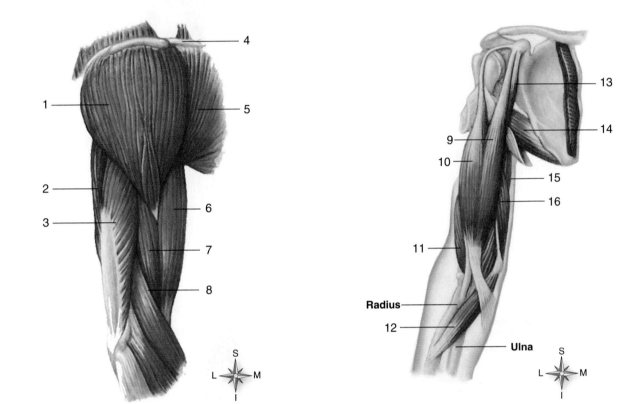

Figure 7.6a

Relevant Terms		
_____ Biceps brachii (long head)	_____ Clavicle	_____ Teres major
_____ Biceps brachii (long head)	_____ Coracobrachialis	_____ Triceps brachii (lateral head)
_____ Biceps brachii (short head)	_____ Deltoid	_____ Triceps brachii (long head)
_____ Brachialis	_____ Pectoralis major	_____ Triceps brachii (long head)
_____ Brachialis	_____ Pronator teres	_____ Triceps brachii (medial head)
_____ Brachioradialis		

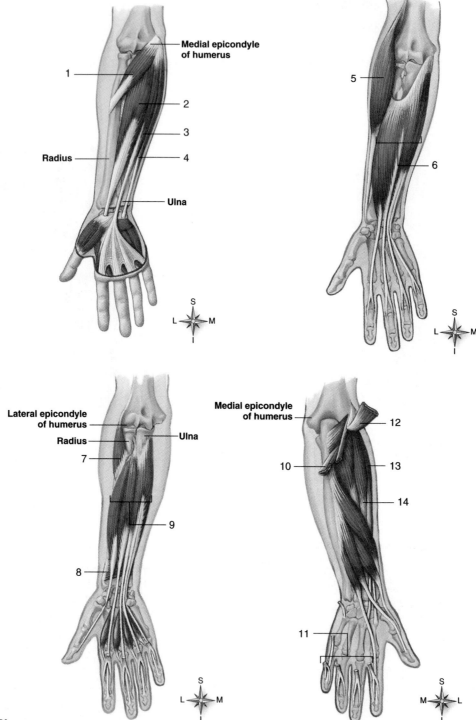

Figure 7.6b

Relevant Terms		
_____ Brachioradialis	_____ Extensor digitorum (cut)	_____ Palmaris longus
_____ Extensor carpi radialis brevis	_____ Flexor digitorum profundis	_____ Pronator quadratus
_____ Extensor carpi radialis longus	_____ Flexor digitorum superficialis	_____ Pronator teres
_____ Extensor carpi ulnaris	_____ Flexor carpi radialis	_____ Supinator
_____ Extensor digitorum (cut)	_____ Flexor carpi ulnaris	

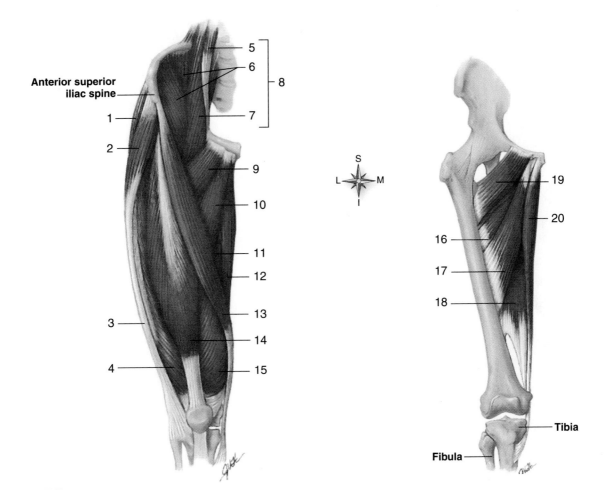

Anterior superior iliac spine

Figure 7.7a

Relevant Terms		
____ Adductor brevis	____ Gracilis	____ Psoas minor
____ Adductor longus	____ Iliacus	____ Rectus femoris
____ Adductor longus	____ Iliopsoas	____ Sartorius
____ Adductor magnus	____ Iliotibial tract	____ Tensor fasciae latae
____ Adductor magnus	____ Pectinius	____ Vastus lateralis
____ Gluteus medius	____ Pectinius	____ Vastus medialis
____ Gracilis	____ Psoas major	

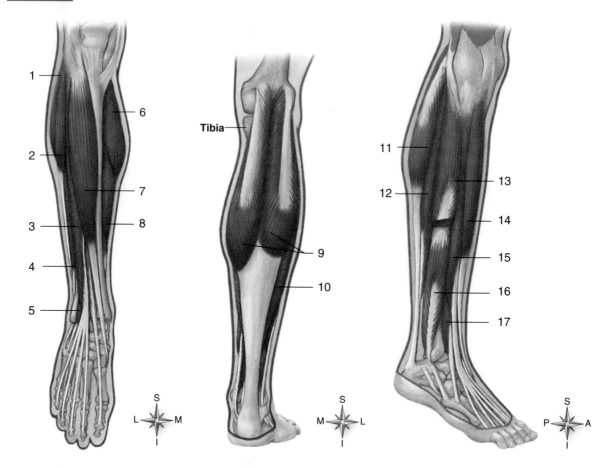

Figure 7.7b

Relevant Terms		
_____ Extensor digitorum longus	_____ Peroneum (fibularis) brevis	_____ Soleus
_____ Extensor digitorum longus	_____ Peroneum (fibularis) longus	_____ Soleus
_____ Gastrocnemius	_____ Peroneum (fibularis) longus	_____ Soleus
_____ Gastrocnemius	_____ Peroneum (fibularis) tertius	_____ Soleus
_____ Gastrocnemius	_____ Peroneum (fibularis) tertius	_____ Tibialis anterior
_____ Peroneum (fibularis) brevis		

Section B. Assessments

1. T/F   The triceps brachii extend the lower arm.
2. T/F   The gastrocnemius extends the thigh.
3. The flexor digitorum profundus is found in which part of the upper extremities?
   a. shoulder
   b. upper arm
   c. lower arm
   d. hand
4. Which of the following is NOT a muscle located in the foot?
   a. lumbricals
   b. abductor hallucis
   c. soleus
   d. all of the above are located in the foot
5. How many muscles are part of the hamstring group?
   a. 1
   b. 2
   c. 3
   d. 4
   e. 5

Section C. Critical Thinking Problems

1. Communication is a vital human activity. Spoken languages are possible because of the muscles that control the mouth, while the muscles of the hands have allowed us to develop sign languages with extremely large vocabularies. Nonverbal communication is important in both spoken and sign languages. What can the hands and face do similarly that allows for their use in communication?

2. Baseball players, particularly pitchers, often incur rotator cuff injuries. List the muscles that make up the rotator cuff and explain the importance of these muscles and their role in joint stability.

Exercise 8

The Integrated Musculoskeletal System

Lesson Overview

Activity #1: Range of Motion

Overview

Determining what is going on inside the human body is a lot like unraveling a superhero's secret identity. Comic book readers know that Spiderman and Peter Parker are the same person. In fact, we gain insight into both sides of his personality by understanding conflicts that each side encounters. In a related way, we have looked under the skin at the musculoskeletal system, separating the two systems to understand each. But just as you can't have the superhero without the alter-ego, neither the skeletal system nor the muscular system could function without its partner.

To finalize our study of the musculoskeletal system, we will survey the variety of motions that are possible once the musculoskeletal system is allowed to kick into action.

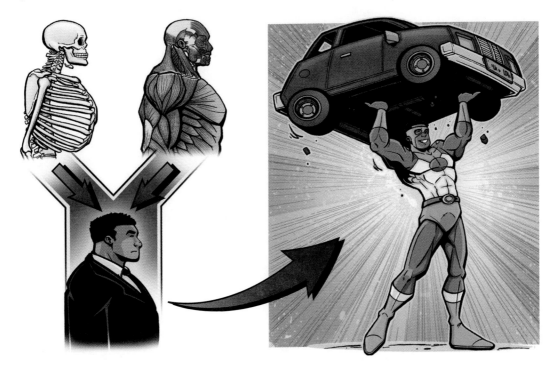

Activity #1 — Range of Motion

Introduction

Superheroes amaze us with their abilities to do incredible things, but their physical prowess is just an exaggeration of what the average person's body can potentially do. True, their bodies are conditioned for strength, agility, and speed, but the range of motion possible cannot be that different, considering we all have the same bipedal body plan.

In light of this, and to fully appreciate the capacity of the integrated musculoskeletal system, we will investigate the range of motion possible by the human body. Now we understand the underlying anatomical structures that allow these motions. Whether we observe crawling toddlers, spinning gymnasts, or The Flash in action, we are witnessing the amazing motion of our own bodies.

Materials

Textbook
Previous models used to study skeletal and muscular systems

Procedure

1. Review content in your textbook related to range of motion.
2. When possible, orient your own body into the positions described. Correlate each position with the type of joints, bones, and muscles that are directly involved in each movement according to both the three-dimensional models and diagrams from your textbook.
3. Identify the various movements possible at synovial joints in Figure 8.2.

Lab Report for 8.1

Section A. Activities for Range of Motion

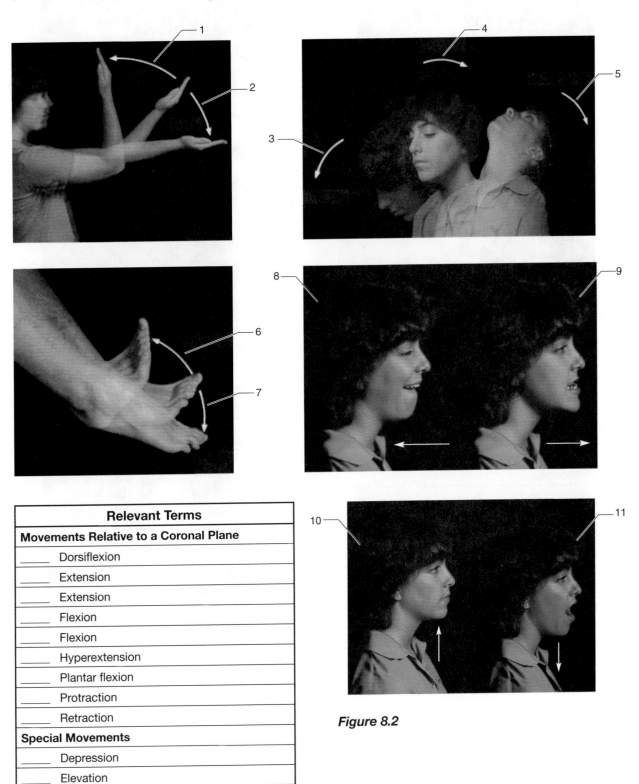

Figure 8.2

Relevant Terms
Movements Relative to a Coronal Plane
_____ Dorsiflexion
_____ Extension
_____ Extension
_____ Flexion
_____ Flexion
_____ Hyperextension
_____ Plantar flexion
_____ Protraction
_____ Retraction
Special Movements
_____ Depression
_____ Elevation

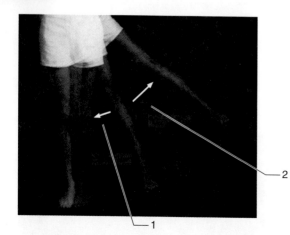

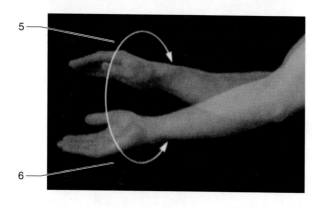

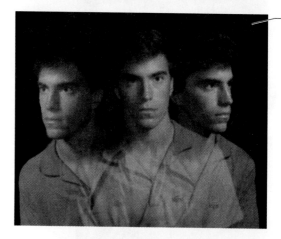

Relevant Terms
Movements Relative to a Coronal Plane
_____ Abduction
_____ Adduction
_____ Eversion
_____ Inversion
Circular Movements
_____ Circumduction
_____ Pronation
_____ Rotation
_____ Supination

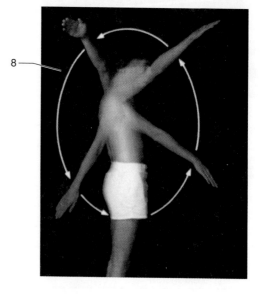

Figure 8.2 (con't)

Section B. Assessments

1. T/F An example of abduction is raising your arm laterally away from your body.
2. T/F Dorsiflexion allows a ballerina to stand on her toes.
3. T/F Moving your hand from a pronated to a supinated position requires rotation of the forearm.
4. Moving a part of the body toward the midline of the body is called:
   a. adduction.
   b. abduction.
   c. rotation.
   d. pronation.
5. The opposite of eversion of the foot is:
   a. plantar flexion.
   b. rotation.
   c. dorsiflexion.
   d. inversion.

Section C. Critical Thinking Problems

1. Imagine a plastic surgeon begins to offer "range of motion" enhancements, providing athletes with greater flexibility.
   a. What might the surgeon do to enhance range of the motion in the back? The arms? The feet?

   b. What possible negative consequences might arise from these enhancements?

2. One notable superhero who is capable of a much wider range of motion than humans is Mr. Fantastic, who is able to stretch his body many different ways. How would human tissue have to be different in order to permit this range of motion?

Unit 3

Communication, Control, and Integration

Deckard: *She's a replicant, isn't she?*

Dr. Tyrell: *I'm impressed. How many questions does it usually take to spot them?*

Deckard: *...twenty, thirty, cross-referenced.*

Dr. Tyrell: *It took more than a hundred for Rachael, didn't it?*

Blade Runner (1982)

Will machines be indistinguishable from humans in the future?

Throughout history, the notion of creating machines to mimic humans has tantalized the imagination. For example, in Greek mythology, the god of craftsmanship, Hephaestus, invented female automatons to assist him in his workshop. Modern science fiction stories and films, such as *Blade Runner*, imagine a world populated with androids. In the 1982 film, a dangerous group of human-like robotic machines called *replicants*, banned from the planet because of an uprising, return to Earth to seek an extension on their four-year life span. These androids are hunted down by a blade runner, a police-hired assassin named Deckard, in an effort to 'retire' them; that is, terminate them. Though Deckard could easily identify old replicants, a new, more human prototype named Rachael was developed that posed a challenge. The film hits upon a popular theme in science fiction: the tantalizing idea that technology could advance to the point that an android would be indistinguishable from a human being.

The complexity of such a technological breakthrough is challenging on multiple levels. It isn't enough for something to merely look human — artists and designers have already made great strides in creating human-looking figures out of various materials. For androids to become a reality they must think, behave, and relate in human ways to such an extent that it would take elaborate tests to determine that they were not human beings.

To appreciate what must be accomplished to achieve such a modern marvel, we must unravel the systems responsible for cognition, behavior, and social interactions that androids must emulate in order to effectively pass as human. Toward this end, we will investigate the nervous system, which is responsible for rapid communication in the body, and the endocrine system, which regulates and controls the body over time.

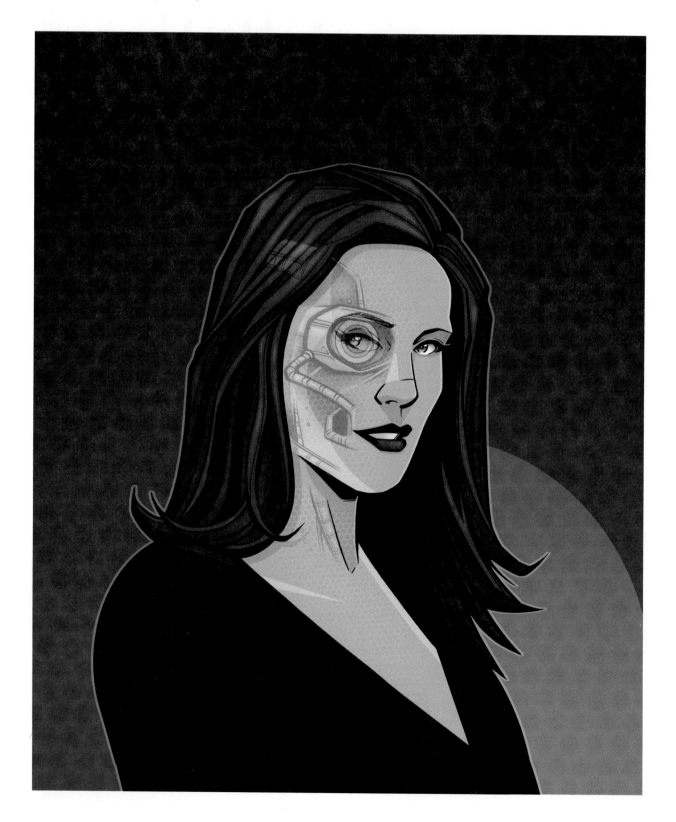

Exercise 9

The Nervous System

Lesson Overview

Activity #1: Neurons and Nerve Tissue
Activity #2: Organization of the Nervous System and Nerve Reflexes
Activity #3: The Central Nervous System (CNS)
  Part A: The Brain
  Part B: The Spinal Cord
Activity #4: The Peripheral Nervous System (PNS)
  Part A: Cranial Nerves
  Part B: Spinal Nerves

Overview

As rapid developments in robotics and artificial intelligence (AI) transform our culture, the twenty-first century will likely involve the adoption of a wide range of thinking machines into many aspects of society. The use of basic robots that perform menial tasks, much like the popular *Roomba*® vacuuming robot, is sure to increase while more social humanoid machines will begin to become more prominent in certain venues, such as tour guides in museums. Although robots akin to the "droids" in *Star Wars*, for instance, would be able to meet many people's needs, androids that look and act human are more socially palatable and could be easily adopted into modern society because of their humanoid designs. Humanness, then, is more than just appearance — everything from facial expressions to nonverbal communication. This involves behavior, including what androids talk about, when they interact, and how they respond to people — all of which are controlled by the nervous system in human beings.

To begin the study of the nervous system, we will first investigate the cellular basis of communication in the body by examining nerves and reflexes. Then we will systematically study the organization of the nervous system, including the brain, spinal cord, and the nerves that extend throughout the rest of the body.

Activity #1 — Neurons and Nerve Tissue

Introduction

Researchers now recognize that recreating the basic unit of the nervous system, neurons, may be the only way to solve the problem of rapid communication in a humanoid. But to what extent must a synthetic version imitate real nerve tissue?

Like copper wires in circuits, neurons transmit electrical signals; however, they accomplish this through a much more complex process than conduction. Signals are sent through the progressive transport of chemical ions across cell membranes. Between neurons are gaps called *synaptic clefts* that control whether signals progress by converting electrical signals into neurotransmitters, which are released into the cleft. In a way, the synapse is akin to an electronic transistor. Other cells of the nervous system, called *glial cells*, had previously been thought to serve only as insulation for neurons, but more recent research revealed a host of functions these cells play, further complicating both our understanding of the nervous system as well as the ability to mimic it.

To appreciate the challenge that AI engineers face, you will investigate the structure of neurons and nerve tissue.

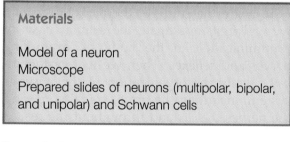

Materials

Model of a neuron
Microscope
Prepared slides of neurons (multipolar, bipolar, and unipolar) and Schwann cells

Procedure

1. Review content in your textbook related to neurons and nervous tissue.
2. Neurons typically conduct impulses or action potentials from dendrites that receive signals from other neurons and propagate these signals into the cell body called the *soma*. The signal continues away from the soma through the axon hillock and into the singular elongated axon until it terminates at synaptic knobs, which are responsible for releasing chemicals called *neurotransmitters* into the synaptic cleft. One type of neuroglial cell, Schwann cells, wrap the axons of neurons in myelin in the brain or spinal cord — that is, neurons that are part of the peripheral nervous system (PNS) — whereas oligodendrocytes wrap the axons of central nervous system (CNS) neurons. Groups of myelinated neurons are called *white matter*, because of the white fatty myelin, while unmyelinated neurons are dubbed *grey matter*. Identify the key structures of a neuron in Figure 9.2.
3. Neurons can be classified into three types. Multipolar neurons, such as motor neurons and many CNS neurons, have structures of the typical neuron described above, with multiple branched dendrites extending from the cell body. Bipolar neurons have only one dendrite attached to the soma and are often found in the nerves of special senses, such as the eyes and ears. Both multiple and bipolar neurons have a single axon that extends from the axon hillock. Unipolar neurons, on the other hand, have only one extension from the cell body, which splits into a dendritic branch and an axon branch. Sensory neurons that transmit to the CNS are commonly unipolar neurons. Examine Figure 9.3 and label the three types of neurons using the terms provided.
4. Besides Schwann cells in the PNS, other types of neuroglia play important functions in the CNS. Astrocytes have elongated projections that attach to blood vessels in the brain, creating a layer that is part of the blood-brain barrier. Ependymal cells both contribute to cerebrospinal fluid as well as line the spaces of the brain and spinal cord that contain this fluid, aiding in fluid flow with cilia. Microglial cells protect the CNS by cleaning up debris and attacking invading pathogens. From the information provided in Figure 9.4, determine the type of glial cell shown.
5. Use the microscope to examine slides of multipolar, bipolar, and unipolar neurons as well as Schwann cells and draw what you observe in your lab report.

Lab Report for 9.1

Section A. Activities for Neurons and Nerve Tissue

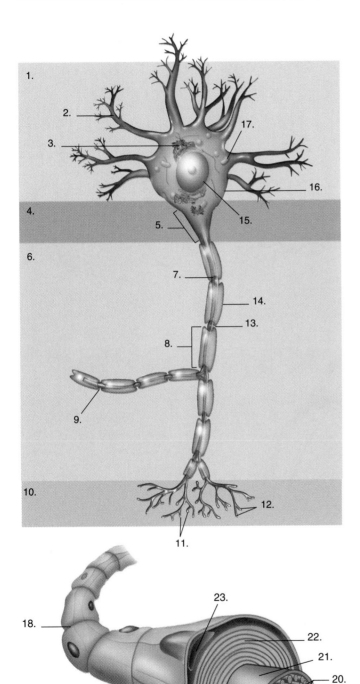

Relevant Terms
_____ Axon
_____ Axon collateral
_____ Axon hillock
_____ Cell body (soma)
_____ Conduction zone
_____ Dendrite
_____ Endoplasmic reticulum
_____ Golgi apparatus
_____ Input zone
_____ Mitochondrion
_____ Myelin sheath
_____ Myelin sheath
_____ Neurilemma (sheath of Schwann cell)
_____ Neurofibrils, microfilaments, and microtubules
_____ Node of Ranvier
_____ Node of Ranvier
_____ Nucleus
_____ Nucleus of Schwann cell
_____ Output zone
_____ Plasma membrane of axon
_____ Schwann cell
_____ Summation zone
_____ Synaptic knobs
_____ Telodendria

Figure 9.2

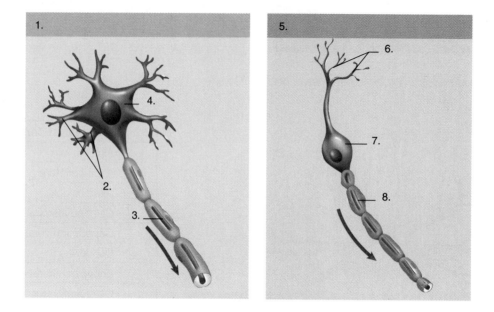

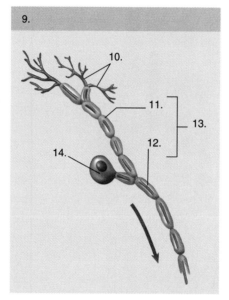

Figure 9.3

Relevant Terms	
_____ Axon	_____ Central process
_____ Axon	_____ Dendrites
_____ Axon	_____ Dendrites
_____ Cell body	_____ Dendrites
_____ Cell body	_____ Multipolar
_____ Cell body	_____ Peripheral process

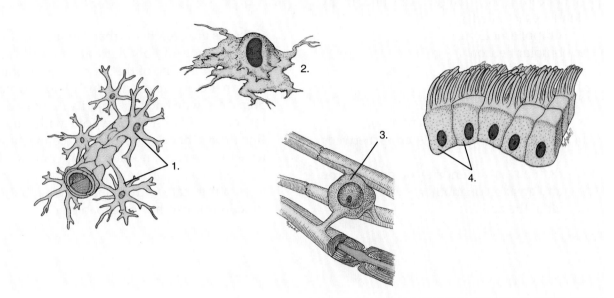

Figure 9.4

Relevant Terms
_____ Astrocytes
_____ Ependymal cells
_____ Microglia
_____ Oligodendrocyte

Draw your observations from prepared slides of neurons and Schwann cells here:

multipolar neurons   bipolar neurons   unipolar neurons   Schwann cells

Section B. Assessments

1. T/F In the PNS, myelin for neurons is produced by Schwann cells.
2. T/F Oligodendrocytes and Schwann cells are similar because they are in the same part of the nervous system, but have quite different functions.

3. Impulses are carried to the cell body of the neuron by which of the following structures?
   a. dendrite
   b. axon
   c. node of Ranvier
   d. axon hillock

4. A neuron with a single axon and many dendrites is called a:
   a. unipolar neuron.
   b. bipolar neuron.
   c. multipolar neuron.
   d. interneuron.
5. The synaptic cleft is:
   a. the gap found between neurons.
   b. point which chemicals cross between neurons.
   c. defined as a dendrite of one neuron and an axon of another.
   d. all of the above.

Section C. Critical Thinking Problem

1. Cyborgs are organisms that contain significant amounts of both natural and artificial components. One of the most recognizable cybernetic organisms is Darth Vader from *Star Wars*, who had the majority of his body (especially his limbs) replaced with functional prosthetics, presumably connecting to actual nerves and not being controlled by the Force. In order for mechanical parts to communicate with a neuron, what basic functions must they be capable of?

Activity #2 — Organization of the Nervous System and Nerve Reflexes

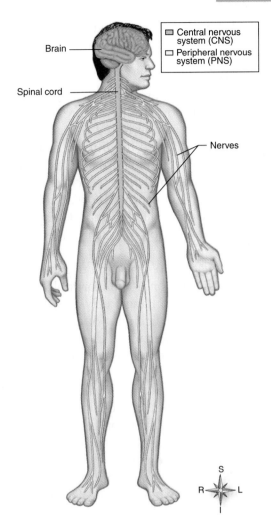

Brain

Spinal cord

Nerves

☐ Central nervous system (CNS)
☐ Peripheral nervous system (PNS)

Introduction

Considering the human nervous system, we may draw some loose parallels to the internal structure of a computer. The brain is the body's CPU, communicating through the spinal cord to the muscles and sensory systems that interact with the environment. Some of these peripheral components spread throughout the body have their own kind of firmware (a type of software encoded in computer components) called *reflex arcs* regulating somatic reflexes, which involve stimulation of skeletal muscle, and autonomic reflexes, which are responsible for regulating many of the internal organ systems, such as heart rate, digestion and sweating.

We can imagine that as engineers seek to build androids, commonalities between computers and the nervous system will be retained, as the entire android is one large, walking, talking computer.

The following activities provide an overview of the nervous system and an investigation into the nerve reflexes present throughout the human body.

Materials

Rubber mallet or hammer
Dim flashlight

Before You Begin

- *While testing reflexes on your partner, it is important that you do not hit too hard with the mallet or strike a bone. Check the spot you are going to strike first to ensure that it is the correct location.*
- *While having your reflexes tested, it is important that you relax the muscles in the region being tested to avoid injury.*

Procedure

1. Review content in your textbook related to overview of the nervous system and reflex arcs.
2. A reflex arc is a way of describing communication of nerve signals or action potentials. In a reflex arc, an input/output program is biologically encoded to transmit a signal produced from a stimulated skin receptor; for instance, through a sensory neuron to an integration center in the spinal cord. This is the afferent neuron. In the spinal cord, the signal may be transmitted directly to an efferent neuron, which communicates with an effector that may contract a muscle or activate a gland. This is an example of a two-neuron or monosynaptic arc. In a three-neuron (polysynaptic) arc, an interneuron is present in the spinal

cord. Label the key structural features of the polysynaptic reflex arc in Figure 9.6.

Stretch Reflexes

3. Stretch reflexes are monosynaptic reflexes that are important in posture and locomotion and can be tested by tapping the tendon attached to the muscle being considered, which will cause a reflex contraction. Test the following stretch reflexes on a partner and record your observations for each reflex in your lab report. Figure 9.7 shows the location for each of the reflexes to be tested.

   a. *Patellar (knee-jerk) reflex*: Have your partner sit on a chair or table that allows legs to hang freely. Gently strike the patellar ligament of each knee below the patella, which will stimulate the quadriceps muscle causing extension of the leg.

   b. *Calcaneal (ankle-jerk) reflex*: Have your partner kneel on a chair such that the toes point to the floor. Gently strike the calcaneal (Achilles) tendon to induce plantar flexion of the foot.

   c. *Biceps reflex*: Have your partner sit and place an exposed arm at a 90-degree angle on a table. Place your thumb on the biceps (brachii) tendon located in the inside of the elbow and press gently. Gently strike your thumb to induce flexion or a slight twitch of the biceps.

   d. *Triceps reflex*: Have your partner lie on a table with an arm bent at a 90-degree angle across the abdomen. Gently strike the triceps (brachii) tendon proximal to the olecranon, which will cause extension of the arm or a slight twitch of the triceps.

Cutaneous Reflexes

4. *Plantar reflex*: Unlike the stretch reflexes that involve striking a tendon, some reflexes can be induced by stimulation of the skin (cutaneous receptors), as shown in Figure 9.7. Have your partner remove shoes and socks and rest the foot to be tested on a lateral surface. Sweep the handle of the mallet over the lateral region of the sole (from the sole to the base of the large toe). Flexion of the toes should occur along with plantar flexion of the foot. In infants, a Babinski reflex is common, in which the toes move apart or the big toe extends.

Cranial Reflexes

5. *Pupillary reflex*: Cranial reflexes are those that relate to the cranial nerves, which may be checked during a routine examination. To properly test the pupillary reflex, conduct the test in a dimly lit area. Have a partner stare straight ahead with one hand shielding the right eye. Shine a dim flashlight into your partner's left eye and determine whether there is any change in pupil size. Also, determine whether the right eye experiences a consensual reflex; that is, a corresponding change in pupil diameter even though light was not shined into it. Repeat the procedure for the right eye.

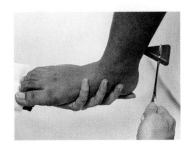

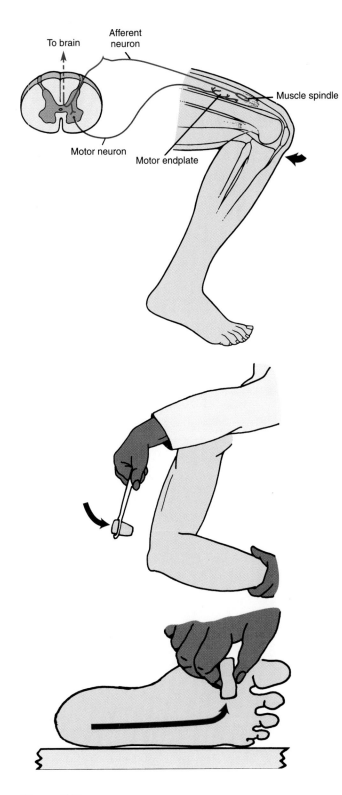

To brain

Afferent
neuron

Muscle spindle

Motor neuron

Motor endplate

Figure 9.7

Lab Report for 9.2

Section A. Organization of the Nervous System and Nerve Reflexes

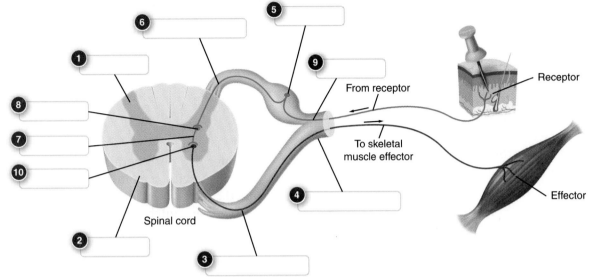

Figure 9.6

Relevant Terms	
Cell body	Sensory neuron axon
Dendrite	Spinal nerve
Gray matter	Synapse
Interneuron	Synapse
Motor neuron axon	White matter

Observations on reflexes

Patellar reflex: _____

_____

Calcaneal reflex: _____

_____

Biceps reflex: _____

_____

Triceps reflex: _____

_____

Plantar reflex: _____

_____

Pupillary reflex: _____

_____

Section B. Assessments

1. T/F   An interneuron must be present in a two-neuron arc.
2. T/F   Motor nerves contain mostly efferent fibers.
3. Impulses are carried away from the CNS by which of the following neurons?
    a. sensory neurons
    b. motor neurons
    c. afferent neurons
    d. both b and c
4. Reflexes involve:
    a. one neuron.
    b. two neurons.
    c. three neurons.
    d. both b and c above.
5. When the outer sole of an infant's foot is stimulated, the toes will extend or spread apart. This is known as the _____ reflex.
    a. corneal
    b. Babinski
    c. pupillary
    d. plantar

Section C. Critical Thinking Problems

1. Taking a cursory glance at how the nervous system is wired throughout the body, would there be an advantage to a cyborg that had a split spinal cord that extended down through each leg?

2. A printer is a peripheral device that communicates with a computer and is controlled by the operating system, but it also has a power switch, which means that outside the computer's control, communication between the two can be cut off when the power is cut. Is an analogous process in neural reflexes possible?

Activity #3 — The Central Nervous System (CNS)

Part A: The Brain

Introduction

Personality. Creativity. Intelligence. Emotion. Sociability. Communication. Morality.

Each of these words captures a complex set of rich behaviors that contribute to our humanness, the seat of which lies within the brain. While these higher-order characteristics often take the limelight, the brain concurrently manages a vast array of the body's inner workings, enabling homeostasis and development to proceed beneath the conscious state while processing, selectively storing, and responding to vast quantities of information streaming in from the sensory systems. The specific anatomical and physiological wiring of a number of complex activities managed by the brain remains a mystery, though great efforts are currently underway in the neurosciences to uncover the mind-brain connections.

And herein lies a dilemma for the development of androids. How are researchers to develop an artificial brain when many of the brain's processes are still unknown? Small steps have been taken toward this monolithic goal. For instance, retinal implants wired directly into the brain have allowed the blind to see again, to a degree. AI researchers have developed software that allows computers to be indistinguishable from humans when performing specific tasks. But clearly, it is a long road ahead for neuroscientists and AI researchers alike to discover how the brain functions as a whole.

Materials

Dissectible model of the brain
Anatomical charts of the brain
Human brain or sheep brain
Plastic human brain models with corresponding diagrams

Procedure

1. Review content in your textbook related to the brain.
2. If possible, examine a physical brain or plastic model to correlate the content and images in your textbook and available charts to physical relationships in a model or actual brain.
3. The functionality of the brain is organized into different general regions, but it is not always strictly relegated to those regions. Some functions span across large portions of the brain, others are in isolated structures. To gain a sense of the structure and topography of the brain, differentiate the hemispheres and lobes in Figure 9.8.
4. The largest part of the brain is the cerebrum, which is divided into two hemispheres (right and left) by a longitudinal fissure. The cortex of the cerebrum, or its surface, features large folds of gray matter marked by shallower sulci and deeper fissures. Communication between these two hemispheres is provided by the corpus callosum. Somewhat posterior and inferior to the cerebrum is the cerebellum. In the interior of the brain is the diencephalon, containing the thalamus and hypothalamus, and inferior to the hypothalamus, the midbrain, pons, and medulla oblongata make up the brainstem. Recognize these structural divisions of the brain in Figure 9.9.
5. Because of the sensitive nature of the CNS tissues, layers of membranes called *meninges* protect the CNS by forming a barrier between it and the bones of the axial skeleton. Identify the meninges around the brain in Figure 9.10.

Part B: The Spinal Cord

Introduction

If the brain is the processing hub of information in the body, the spinal cord is the main pipeline for information transfer, like a fiber-optic cable connecting a computer to the Internet. It is much more sophisticated than a simple biological cable, however. Some patients with CNS damage in which the communication between the brain and spinal cord has been compromised have regained the ability to walk. Patients with severe injuries have also regained the ability to walk by using an exoskeleton-like robotic device as part of their physical therapy.

The ability of the spinal cord to function independently of the brain suggests that "learning" may be occurring in the spinal cord itself.

Like the brain, there is still much to learn about the spinal cord. For now, use this activity to increase your knowledge of brain fundamentals.

Materials

Spinal cord model with meninges

Procedure

1. Review content in your textbook related to the spinal cord.
2. Label the structures of the spinal cord and meninges in this cross-section according to Figure 9.11.
3. Identify the 31 pairs of segments in the spinal cord in Figure 9.12.

Lab Report for 9.3

Section A. The Brain

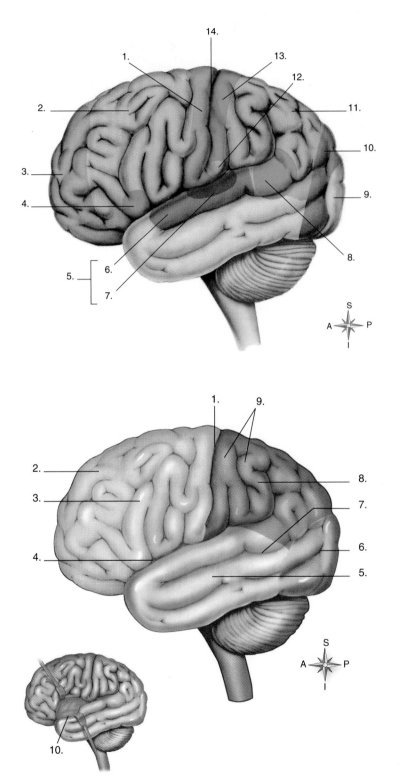

Relevant Terms
Functional Areas
_____ Auditory association area
_____ Central sulcus
_____ Motor speech (Broca) area
_____ Postcentral gyrus (primary somatic sensory area)
_____ Precentral gyrus (primary somatic motor area)
_____ Prefrontal area
_____ Premotor area
_____ Primary auditory area
_____ Primary taste area
_____ Sensory speech (Wernicke) area
_____ Somatic sensory association area
_____ Transverse gyrus
_____ Visual association area
_____ Visual cortex
Left Hemishpere
_____ Central sulcus
_____ Frontal lobe
_____ Insula (Reil island)
_____ Lateral fissure
_____ Occipital lobe
_____ Parietal lobe
_____ Parieto-occipital fissure
_____ Postcentral gyrus
_____ Superior frontal gyrus
_____ Temporal lobe

Figure 9.8

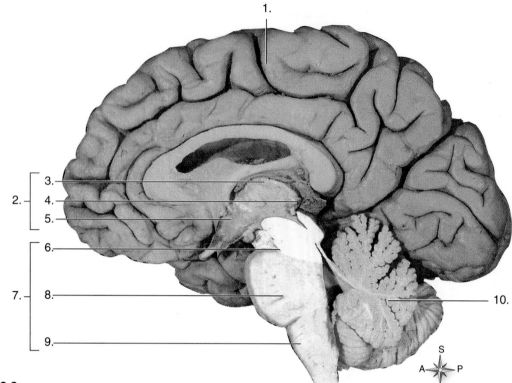

Figure 9.9

Relevant Terms			
_____	Brainstem	_____	Medulla oblongata
_____	Cerebellum	_____	Midbrain
_____	Cerebrum	_____	Pineal body
_____	Diencephalon	_____	Pons
_____	Hypothalamus	_____	Thalamus

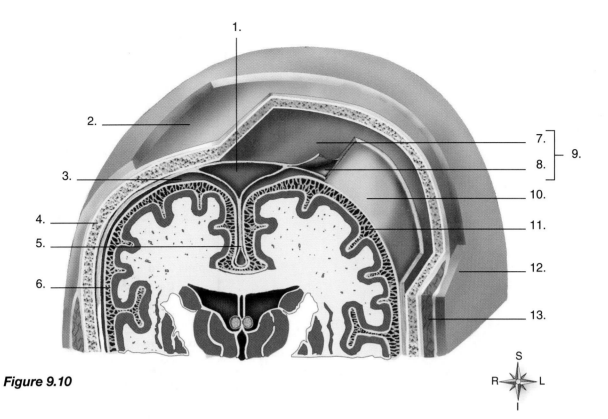

Figure 9.10

Relevant Terms	
_____ Arachnoid mater	_____ Pia mater
_____ Dura mater	_____ Skin
_____ Falx cerebri	_____ Skull
_____ Muscle	_____ Subarachnoid space
_____ One functional layer	_____ Subdural space
_____ Periosteum	_____ Superior sagittal sinus (of dura)
_____ Periosteum	

Section B. The Spinal Cord

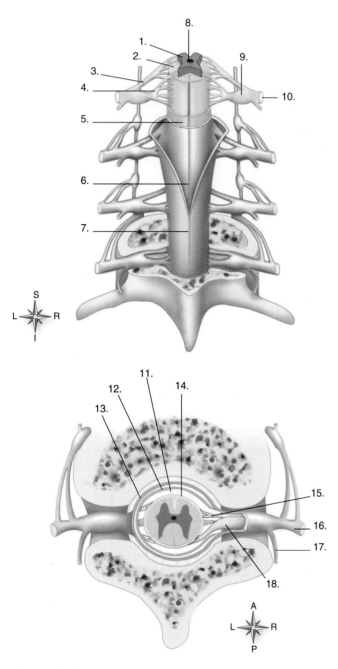

Relevant Terms
Meninges
_____ Arachnoid mater
_____ Arachnoid mater
_____ Dura mater
_____ Dura mater
_____ Pia mater
_____ Pia mater
_____ Subarachnoid space
Spinal Cord
_____ Central canal
_____ Gray matter
_____ White matter
Spinal Nerve
_____ Dorsal ramus
_____ Dorsal root
_____ Dorsal root ganglion
_____ Dorsal root ganglion
_____ Spinal nerve
_____ Ventral ramus
_____ Ventral root
_____ Ventral root

Figure 9.11

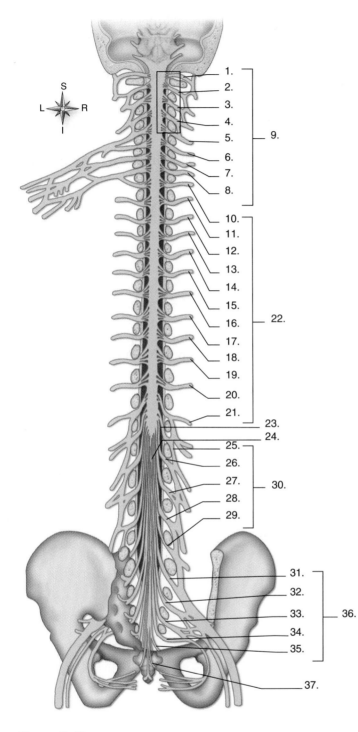

Figure 9.12

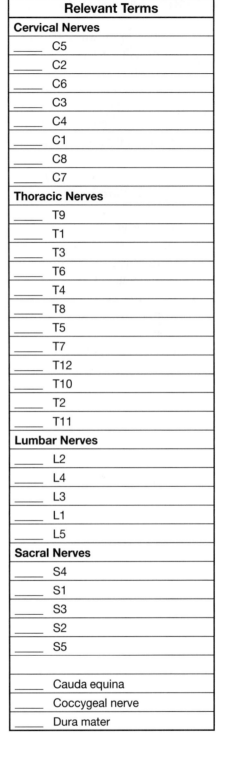

Relevant Terms
Cervical Nerves
_____ C5
_____ C2
_____ C6
_____ C3
_____ C4
_____ C1
_____ C8
_____ C7
Thoracic Nerves
_____ T9
_____ T1
_____ T3
_____ T6
_____ T4
_____ T8
_____ T5
_____ T7
_____ T12
_____ T10
_____ T2
_____ T11
Lumbar Nerves
_____ L2
_____ L4
_____ L3
_____ L1
_____ L5
Sacral Nerves
_____ S4
_____ S1
_____ S3
_____ S2
_____ S5
_____ Cauda equina
_____ Coccygeal nerve
_____ Dura mater

Section C. Assessments

1. T/F   The right and left sides of the brain communicate to each other through the cerebellum.
2. T/F   Sulci are the shallower ridges in the cerebral cortex.
3. T/F   The visual association area is in the occipital lobe of the prefrontal area.
4. Coordination of locomotion and equilibrium is maintained by the:
   a. hypothalamus.
   b. cerebellum.
   c. thalamus.
   d. pons.
5. The outer layer of meninges made of strong fibrous tissue is the:
   a. dura mater.
   b. ventricles.
   c. pia mater.
   d. arachnoid mater.

6. The brainstem includes the:
   a. cerebellum, medulla oblongata, and thalamus.
   b. medulla oblongata, midbrain, and hypothalamus.
   c. hypothalamus, pons, and cerebellum.
   d. medulla oblongata, pons, and midbrain.
7. Which of the following is NOT a lobe of the brain?
   a. temporal lobe
   b. occipital lobe
   c. posterior lobe
   d. frontal lobe

Section D. Critical Thinking Problem

1. How might robotics engineers utilize spinal cord research to build a better android?

Activity #4 — The Peripheral Nervous System (PNS)

Part A: Cranial Nerves

Introduction

Modern computers have an increasing number of components — such as controllers for disk drives and video, sound, and network cards — that at one time were peripheral devices but now are integrated directly onto the motherboard. Furthermore, these components have been miniaturized and can handle more functions, so that today's computers are much more powerful and more self-contained than computers in the past.

Similar to the design of modern motherboards, the CPU-like brain connects to various components in the head, such as sensory organs and muscles. These connections are the cranial nerves, which will be investigated in the following activity. The cranial nerves are part of the peripheral nervous system (PNS), the conduit of information for interacting and engaging with the outside world. In fact, all senses and motor function are part of the PNS, which connects muscles, glands, and sensory systems to the brain and spinal cord.

Materials

Skull, for reference
Cranial nerve model
Spinal cord model, for reference

Procedure

1. Review content in your textbook related to the cranial nerves.
2. Label the cranial nerves according to the information provided in Figure 9.13.

Part B: Spinal Nerves

Introduction

Most computers and cell phones require little maintenance. If androids are ever to make their way into daily life, they too will have to literally take care of themselves along with whatever task they are designed to accomplish.

Likewise, autonomic pathways in the PNS handle an enormous number of tasks automatically. The autonomic nervous system (ANS) connects the brain to organs of the body, via sensory and motor pathways, in order to control and monitor them. The ANS consists of the sympathetic nervous system, which maintains heart rate, blood pressure, and muscle tone as well as the fight-or-flight response. The parasympathetic nervous system controls regular functioning often deemed as rest-and-repair.

In this lab, you will be determining the density of temperature and touch receptors on the skin.

Materials

Diagrams of the nervous system
Nervous system model, if available
Various colored washable markers
Metals spoons
Hot plates
Beakers
Ice
Calipers

Before You Begin

- *Students should dress appropriately for this lab, specifically clothes that allow them easy access to points on their body to test sense of touch, such as forearms and calves.*
- *Students will need to be teamed into groups of two or three for the following activities.*
- *Metal spoons should be kept in the baths until needed. When they are removed, be sure to dry them to avoid any sensations other than temperature.*
- *When students are being prodded with the spoons, their eyes should remain closed.*

Procedure

1. Review content in your textbook related to the spinal nerves and the autonomic nervous system.
2. Use Figure 9.14 to identify the major organs and pathways of the autonomic nervous system.

Density of Temperature Receptors in the Skin

3. Make a cold (0° C) water bath and warm (40° C) water bath and place a few spoons in each.
4. Draw a 2x2-inch square on the anterior side of the forearm of your partner and another on the posterior side of the calf using a pen. You will create a sensory map that shows locations where you experience the sensations of cold and warm on your skin.
5. Using the ice-cold spoon, softly touch various points within each square on your partner and record cold sensations directly on their skin with a blue pen or on a paper grid corresponding to the skin map.
6. Using the warm spoon, softly touch various points within each square on your partner and record warm sensations directly on their skin with a red pen.
7. Make a copy of the sensory map in your lab report.

Two-Point Threshold Test

8. The two-point threshold test is a technique to determine the density of touch receptors in the skin, which varies depending on body region.
9. Initially with the calipers open wide, softly touch the skin of your partner. Your partner will tell you whether he or she can distinguish the sensation as two points or only one.
10. Reduce the width of the calipers, and again softly touch your partner's skin. Continue to adjust the width until your partner reports being able to feel only one point. It may be necessary to randomize the width to acquire the best results or to use a single point of the caliper.
11. Repeat the measurement three times per location.
12. Record the minimum distance of the caliper at each location. Record the type of skin tested.

Lab Report for 9.4

Section A. Cranial Nerves

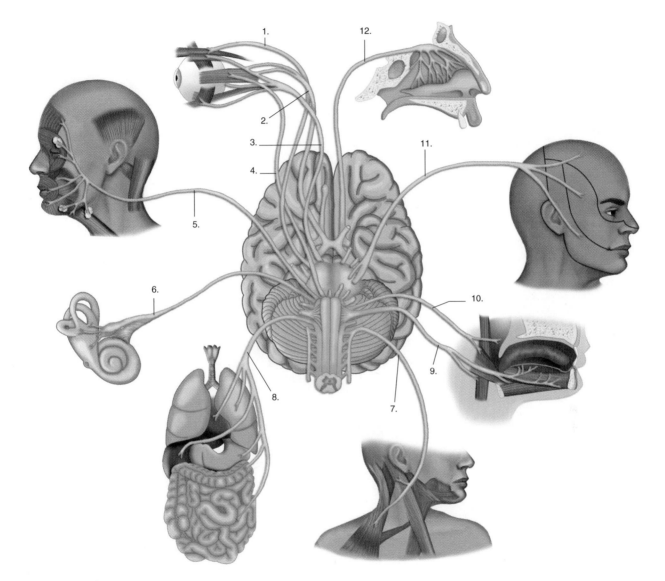

Figure 9.13

Relevant Terms	
_____ Abducens nerve (VI)	_____ Olfactory nerve (I)
_____ Accessory nerve (XI)	_____ Optic nerve (II)
_____ Facial nerve (VII)	_____ Trigeminal nerve (V)
_____ Glossopharyngeal nerve (IX)	_____ Trochlear nerve (IV)
_____ Hypoglossal nerve (XII)	_____ Vagus nerve (X)
_____ Oculomotor nerve (III)	_____ Vestibulocochlear nerve (VIII)

Section B. Spinal Nerves

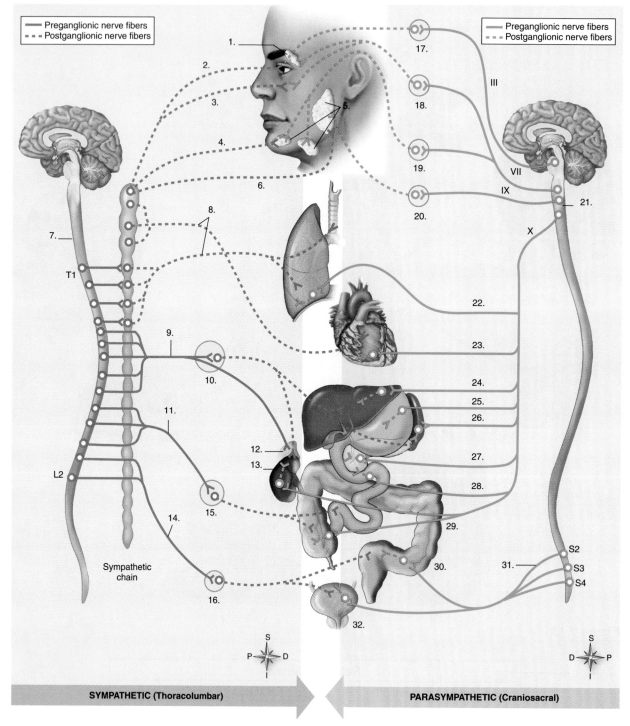

Preganglionic nerve fibers
Postganglionic nerve fibers

Preganglionic nerve fibers
Postganglionic nerve fibers

1.
2.
3.
4.
5.
6.
7.
8.
9.
10.
11.
12.
13.
14.
15.
16.

17.
18.
19.
20.
21.
22.
23.
24.
25.
26.
27.
28.
29.
30.
31.
32.

III
VII
IX
X

T1
L2

Sympathetic chain

S2
S3
S4

S
P — D
I

S
D — P
I

SYMPATHETIC (Thoracolumbar)

PARASYMPATHETIC (Craniosacral)

Figure 9.14

Relevant Terms		
_____ Adrenal gland	_____ Lesser splanchnic nerve	_____ Salivary glands
_____ Celiac ganglion	_____ Liver	_____ Small intestine
_____ Ciliary ganglion	_____ Lumbar splanchnic nerve	_____ Spinal cord
_____ Colon	_____ Lung	_____ Spleen
_____ Eye	_____ Medulla	_____ Stomach
_____ Greater splanchnic nerve	_____ Nasal mucosa	_____ Sublingual and submandibular glands
_____ Heart	_____ Otic ganglion	_____ Submandibular ganglion
_____ Inferior mesenteric ganglion	_____ Pancreas	_____ Superior mesenteric ganglion
_____ Kidney	_____ Parotid gland	_____ Sympathetic nerves
_____ Lacrimal gland	_____ Pelvic nerve	_____ Urinary system and genitalia
_____ Large intestine	_____ Pterygopalatine ganglion	

Density of Temperature Receptors in the Skin: _____

_____

Two-Point Threshold Test: _____

_____

Section C. Assessments

1. T/F The parasympathetic nervous system regulates the "fight-or-flight" response.
2. T/F The nerves of the eyes and ears are considered part of the peripheral nervous system.
3. T/F The autonomic nervous system is less likely to stimulate a voluntary muscle than a smooth muscle.
4. Neurons in the autonomic nervous system conduct impulses from the CNS to:
   a. smooth muscle.
   b. glandular tissue.
   c. cardiac muscle.
   d. all of the above.
5. Altogether, there are _____ cranial nerves.
   a. 5
   b. 12
   c. 24
   d. 31

Section D. Critical Thinking Problem

1. Why would the variation of nerve ending density in the skin be an advantage for the nervous system? Why not have all skin innervated equally?

Exercise 10

The Sensory Systems

Overview

Living things thrive because of their ability to monitor and respond to their external surroundings, often called *adaptation*, while maintaining the stability of their internal environments, which is known as *homeostasis*. In humans, the sensory system and endocrine system carry out these functions in cooperation with the brain. While modern robots demonstrate similar functionalities, they lack the sophistication of these two systems as demonstrated in the average human being.

To begin the study of sensory systems, we will examine the general senses of touch, pain, and pressure within the body. Then we will systematically investigate the special senses of sight, hearing, smell, and taste. In the next exercise, we will consider how the development of robotic devices that need to monitor themselves over the long-term can learn a great deal from the endocrine system.

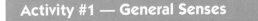
Activity #1 — General Senses

Introduction

Imagine if a museum containing classic works of art had a single temperature sensor and one security camera for the whole building. This severe lack of oversight would most certainly prove disastrous, either because thieves could walk in and take what they wanted or because the lack of proper temperature and humidity controls would destroy the art. Priceless art must be in a carefully controlled environment that is constantly under surveillance with sensors and cameras distributed throughout the museum.

The body has similar control systems, collectively termed the *general senses*, for monitoring both the internal and external environments. The general senses can be further divided into somatic and visceral senses. Somatic senses relate to tactile (touch), thermal, and pain sensations along the skin and proprioceptive sensations, which provide information about the position and motion of the parts of the body relative to one another; proprioceptive sensations help you determine if you are right side up or upside down. Visceral senses monitor the internal environment with receptors along organs.

In this activity, you will explore somatic senses to better understand the distribution of sensory receptors throughout the body.

Materials

Diagrams or models of the skin, including cutaneous receptors
Washable pens and markers
Ruler
Coins
Stopwatch
Bowls
Ice
Rubber mallet

Before You Begin

- Be sure to wear appropriate clothing, such as shorts, for the experiments on sensations.

Procedure

1. Review the section in your textbook related to the general senses.

Locating Tactile Sensations

2. Draw a 2x2-inch square with a washable pen on two or more of the following sites on your partner: the back of the hand, the top of the foot, the ventral side of the forearm, and/or on the thigh just above the patella.

3. With your partner's eyes closed, touch a spot in the square with a marker of a particular color. Have your partner attempt to touch the same spot with a different colored marker. Measure the distance between the two marks and record the distance.

4. Repeat this measurement at least three times for each site selected.

Sensory Adaptation to Touch

5. With your partner's eyes closed, place a coin on the anterior surface of the forearm and start recording the time that the sensation lasts. When your partner can no longer feel the sensation of the coin, record the amount of time that has elapsed. Leave the coin in this spot.

6. Repeat step #5 with two coins and then three coins at separate locations of the forearm.

7. Add two coins to the original coin in step #5 and record the amount of time until the sensation is lost.

Sensory Adaptation to Temperature

8. Prepare three bowls: one filled with ice water, the second with warm water (40-45° C), and the third with room-temperature water (around 22° C).

9. Have your partner place his or her left hand in the ice water and right hand in the warm water. Record the different sensations as described by your partner.

10. After 2 minutes, have your partner place both hands into the bowl of room-temperature water. Record the different sensations as described by your partner.

Referred Pain: Touch and Temperature

11. Using a rubber mallet, tap the ulnar nerve on your partner's elbow at various locations. Record the different sensations of pain or tingling as described by your partner.

12. Have your partner place the other elbow into the bowl of ice water. Record the different sensations as described by your partner. The sensations will change, so be sure to record his or her observations every 30 seconds or so for two minutes.

13. After two minutes, have your partner remove and dry the elbow. Record the different sensations as described by your partner. The sensations will change, so be sure to record his or her observations every 30 seconds or so for two minutes.

Lab Report for 10.1

Section A. Activities for the General Senses

Record your observations for each of the following activities:

Locating tactile sensations: _____

_____

_____

Sensory adaptation to touch: _____

_____

_____

Sensory adaptation to temperature: _____

_____

_____

Referred pain: Touch and temperature: _____

_____

_____

Section B. Assessments

1. T/F   Sensations involve the conversion of physical stimuli into nerve impulses.
2. T/F   General sense organs are almost exclusively found in the internal organs.
3. General sense receptors are most prevalent in:
   a. internal organs.
   b. muscle tissue.
   c. the skin.
   d. bones.
4. Which of the following sensations is NOT a somatic sense?
   a. touch
   b. pain
   c. pressure
   d. sight

Section C. Critical Thinking Problem

1. Part of the sense of touch is the stimulation of hairs, both when they are pushed down and when they spring back. Would something akin to hairs be valuable for an android to monitor its environment?

Activity #2 — Special Senses

Part A: Visual System

Introduction

One of the key ways we recognize people is by the details of their faces. Toward this end, the human brain becomes highly active during facial perception. While the collection of visual data depends on wavelengths and intensity of light striking the retina in the eye, the sense of vision occurs in the brain. Facial recognition software, used for surveillance and security, must mimic the way the human brain interprets visual information.

The human visual system is particularly good at pattern recognition and is sensitive to a wide range of lighting conditions. In addition, the human visual system achieves upwards of 500 megapixel resolution and image processing speeds under 150 ms. But visual processing in the brain involves more than just passively waiting for the flow of signals from the optic nerve. For instance, research suggests that optical illusions are attempts by the brain to anticipate how elements of an image are changing position, indicating that the visual system is hard-wired to make predictions. In other words, illusions on paper or even by magicians manipulate the brain, not the eye. Clearly there is more to "seeing" than just opening your eyes.

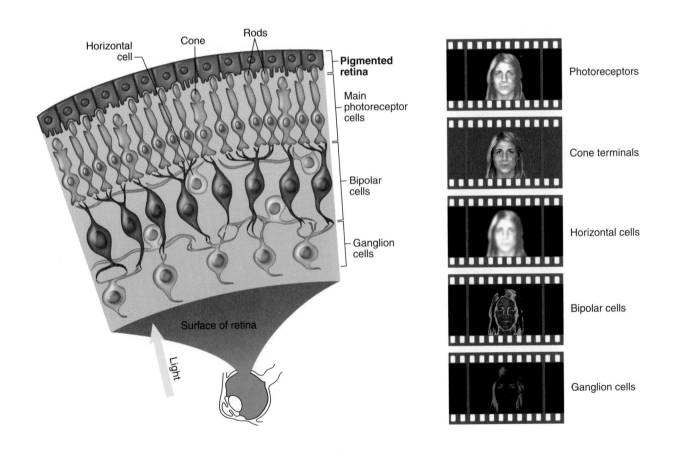

Materials

Diagrams or models of the eye
Dissectible model eye
Index cards
Black markers
Snellen eye chart

Procedure

1. Review the section in your textbook related to the visual system.

Anatomy of the Visual System

2. While referencing a diagram of the eye or the model, identify the external structures and the muscles of the eye according to Figure 10.2 in the Lab Report.
3. Determine the various structures in the layers of the eye as shown in Figure 10.3 in the Lab Report.

Blind Spot

4. There is a portion of the visual field in each eye about which the brain is constantly lying to us: the blind spot. This is the point in the visual field where the optic nerve is located and attaches to the retina; hence, there are no photoreceptors and the brain fabricates the lost information by composing a false image with information from the surrounding visual field.
5. To identify the blind spot, draw a dot and an '+,' each about the size of a pea, on an index card, spaced apart by about 10 cm as shown in Figure 10.4.
6. Hold the index card at arm's length. With your non-testing eye closed and your testing eye focused on the '+', slowly bring the index card closer to your face. At a point typically less than 30 cm, the dot will disappear as its image falls on your optic nerve. It disappears because your brain fills in that missing visual information with what it observes around the blind spot. Record the distance.
7. Once you identify the blind spot, you can attempt to move the index card back and forth at an angle such that the dot is never visible.

Figure 10.4

Visual Acuity Test

8. Use a Snellen eye chart to test the clearness of vision of your partner. Have your partner stand about 6 meters from the chart and cover one eye. Have your partner read each row, starting from the top row. For those who wear glasses, conduct the test twice, once with glasses on and once off. Record the acuity in each of his or her eyes for reference.

Color Blindness Test

9. View the color images in Figure 10.5 while holding them at arm's length. Allow only a few seconds to determine what the number is. Record any discrepancies in your lab report.

Afterimages

10. Afterimages are false images that are visible after photoreceptors are stimulated repeatedly and become fatigued or desensitized — in effect, the photoreceptors are bleached. When the image is removed and replaced with a white background, the least fatigued receptors become more active then the depleted ones, which produces the afterimage.

11. Stare at the '+' in each of the images in Figure 10.6 for 30-60 seconds, and either close your eyes or immediately stare at a blank sheet of paper. It may take a few seconds for the afterimage to be resolvable. Record your observations.

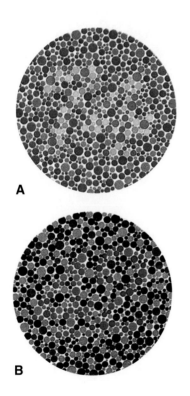

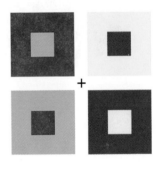

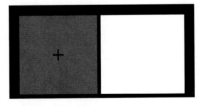

Figure 10.5

Figure 10.6

Optical Illusions

12. Observe the optical illusions in Figure 10.7 and describe the perceived motion of each. Because of the particular patterns in the illusion, the brain anticipates the motion of the shapes even though the image is static.

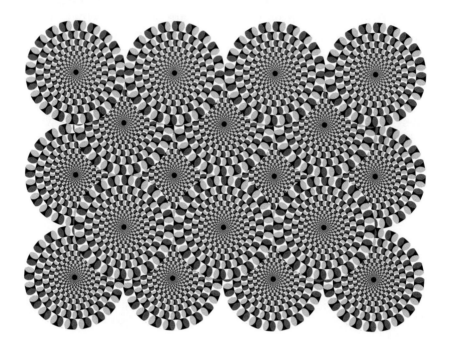

Figure 10.7

Part B: Auditory System

Introduction

Speech recognition software is being increasingly implemented in cell phones and utilized in calling centers. But if speech recognition was the only challenge facing AI engineers developing androids, the development of robotic auditory systems would be trivial compared to the problem of vision. The sense of hearing is much more complex than speech recognition alone. The human auditory system can hone in on specific sounds in a sea of noise and span a range of 20-20,000 Hertz. The auditory signals the ears receive actually undergo significant processing before they are sent to the brain, including amplification. In a sense, the bony structures of the inner ear are a biological answer to advanced digital processing of audio signals, for which software that mimics some of the ear's capabilities has already been developed.

These functions present a challenge to researchers, especially because much of the focus in artificial sensory systems has been on mimicking the visual system. To appreciate the intricacies of the sense of hearing, you will investigate both the anatomy and function of the auditory system.

Materials

Model of the ear
Cotton balls
Tuning forks
Analog watch or stopwatch that audibly ticks
Meter stick

Procedure

1. Review the section in your textbook related to the auditory system.
2. Identify the major structures of the ear in Figure 10.8 in the Lab Report.
3. Identify the structures of the inner ear in Figure 10.9 in the Lab Report.

Rinne Test
4. The Rinne test is a method of comparing the perception of sound as it is conducted through air versus bone and thus helps identify hearing loss.
5. Strike a tuning fork and the place the handle against your partner's mastoid process, as shown in Figure 10.10.
6. When your partner no longer hears the tuning fork, hold the vibrating prongs near your partner's auditory canal. Your partner should report hearing the hum again, which passes via air conduction.

7. Repeat on the other side of the head.
8. Repeat steps 3-5 but reverse the order, allowing your partner to hear the sound via air conduction first, then once it is no longer heard, placing the handle on your partner's mastoid process.

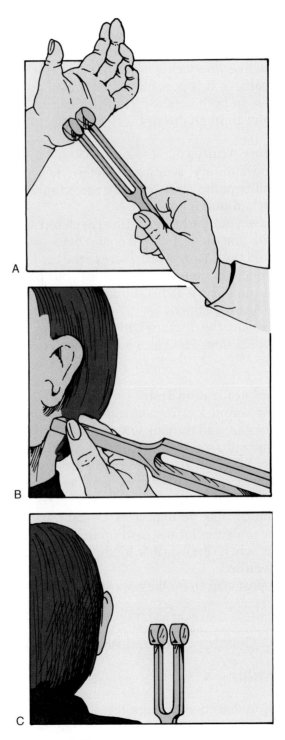

Figure 10.10

Weber Test

9. The Weber test determines if hearing is balanced between the two ears or is lateralized to one side.

    Strike the tuning fork and place the handle medially on your partner's head (the middle of your partner's forehead).

10. Your partner should indicate if the sound is equally clear in both ears or not. If the sound is noticeably louder or softer in one ear, it may indicate deafness, either conductive (louder) or sensorineural (softer) deafness. It is possible to have equal deafness in both ears, which is difficult to resolve through this test.

Auditory Acuity

11. The auditory acuity test determines the ability of the ear to resolve a sound against background noise.

12. Have your partner sit with eyes closed and with one ear sealed by a cotton ball.

13. Hold the ticking watch close to the ear that is open and move it away from your partner until the watch's sound can no longer be heard distinctly.

14. Measure the distance with a meter stick.

15. Repeat steps 11-13 for your partner's other ear.

Sound Localization Test

16. The sound localization test maps out the areas around the ears within which the location of a sound's source can be identified.

17. Hold the watch about 6 inches from your partner's head. With the partner's eyes still closed, move the watch to various locations. Ask your partner to state where the watch is located and identify any areas where the watch's location cannot be identified.

18. Repeat step 16 for the opposite ear.

Part C: Olfactory and Gustatory Systems

Introduction

Chemical detection through the olfactory system is an important part of human life, serving to warn us of a threat, such as a natural gas leak or something burning. In social interactions, the sense of smell can be advantageous, whether it aids in finding a mate or promotes bonding between a newborn and mother. But much of what we smell can't be directly correlated to issues of survival. The perfume industry, for instance, is a testament to the complexity and subtleness that the human nose can sense, yet the ability to smell a breadth of fragrances is not necessarily essential for living. Similarly, the gustatory system, which provides the sense of taste, helps us to avoid eating food that is rotten or potentially poisonous, but the human palate is capable of discerning a variety of tastes beyond what would necessarily be required to identify harmful food.

Both the olfactory and gustatory systems demonstrate the aesthetic quality of human sensation, which presents a perplexing situation for AI researchers: Is there any aesthetic value in the senses for robots and androids? It seems reasonable that if an android is to be a true replica of a human being, it should know beyond trivial knowledge why certain foods are unappetizing while others smell good and taste delicious. Furthermore, the taste of food is heavily influenced by its smell. Both of these systems function through chemical detection of specific substances, and hence compound the challenge to artificial systems for smell and taste.

> **Materials**
>
> Model of the nose
> Model of the tongue
> Stopwatch
> Blue food coloring
> Paper towels
> Cotton swab
> Hole punch
> Hand lens

Procedure

1. Review the section in your textbook related to the olfactory and gustatory systems.

Sense of Smell

2. Identify the major structures of the nose in Figure 10.11 in the Lab Report.
3. Test the ability to identify different smells. First, collect a few bottled samples that your instructor has provided. While your partner's eyes are closed, pass the sample underneath the nose by at least a few inches and ask him or her to identify the odor. Write down the responses in your notebook and continue with the next sample.

Sense of Taste

4. Identify the major structures of the gustatory system in Figure 10.12 in the Lab Report.
5. Using a mirror, identify the different papillae on your own tongue.
6. Dry the surface of your tongue with a paper towel and properly dispose of the towel.

7. Place a few crystals of salt on your tongue and time how long it takes before you can taste the salt.
8. Repeat step 9 using sugar crystals instead.
9. Some people can have a higher number of fungiform papillae than others, and therefore experience the sense of taste with much greater intensity than others. They are collectively dubbed *supertasters* and this can be an underlying cause of picky eating, especially if they report not liking the taste of raw broccoli and preferring salty foods (which may help to reduce the intensity of other flavors present).
10. To visually identify the number of papillae on the tongue, first punch a hole with the hole punch in a small piece of paper. This will be a viewing window for you to count your partner's papillae.
11. Your partner will dry the tongue with a paper towel. Place a drop of blue food coloring on a cotton swab and cover the surface of your partner's tongue with the dye.
12. Place the paper on the tongue so that the center of the tip of the tongue is exposed through the hole. In the presence of a good light source, count the number of pink papillae in the hole. On average, supertasters will have between around 30 papillae. In a taster, 15-30 are present, while people with less than 15 papillae are dubbed *non-tasters*. Non-tasters often prefer food that is sweeter.

Lab Report for 10.2

Section A. Activities for the Visual System

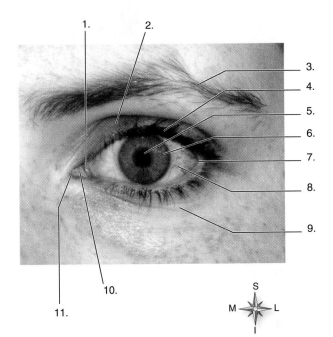

Relevant Terms
_____ Eyebrow
_____ Eyelashes
_____ Inferior oblique
_____ Iris
_____ Lacrimal caruncle
_____ Lateral angle (canthus)
_____ Lateral rectus
_____ Levator palpebrae superioris (cut)
_____ Lower (inferior) eyelid
_____ Medial angle (canthus)
_____ Medial rectus
_____ Optic nerve
_____ Pupil
_____ Sclera
_____ Semilunar fold
_____ Superior oblique
_____ Superior rectus
_____ Trochlea
_____ Upper (superior) eyelid

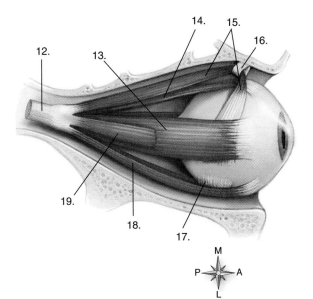

Figure 10.2

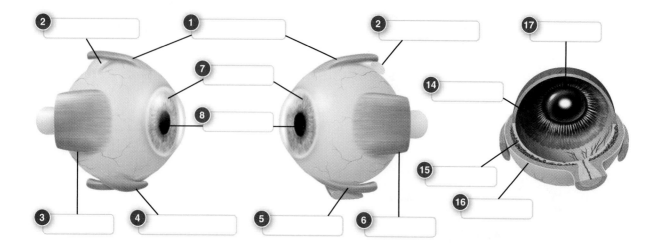

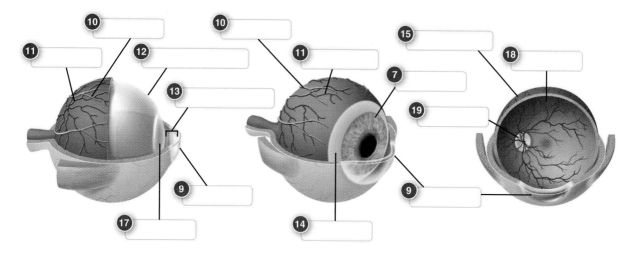

Figure 10.3

Relevant Terms		
Anterior chamber (aqueous humor)	Cornea	Optic disc
Choroid	Cornea	Posterior chamber (vitreous humor)
Choroid	Inferior oblique	Pupil
Ciliary artery	Inferior rectus	Pupil
Ciliary artery	Iris	Retina
Ciliary muscle	Iris	Sclera
Ciliary muscle	Lateral rectus	Sclera
Ciliary nerve	Lens	Superior oblique
Ciliary nerve	Lens	Superior oblique
Cornea	Medial rectus	Superior rectus

Record your observations for each of the following activities:

Blind spot: _____

_____

_____

Visual acuity test: _____

_____

_____

Color blindness test: _____

_____

_____

Afterimages: _____

_____

_____

Optical illusions: _____

_____

_____

Section B. Activities for the Auditory System

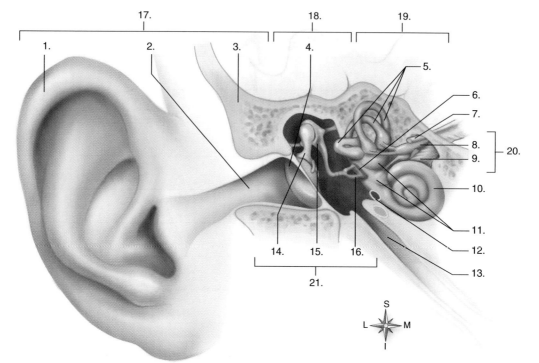

Figure 10.8

Relevant Terms		
_____ Auditory ossicles	_____ Facial nerve	_____ Semicircular canals
_____ Auditory tube	_____ Incus	_____ Stapes
_____ Auricle (pinna)	_____ Inner ear	_____ Temporal bone
_____ Cochlea	_____ Malleus	_____ Tympanic membrane
_____ Cochlear nerve	_____ Middle ear	_____ Vestibular nerve
_____ External acoustic meatus	_____ Oval window	_____ Vestibule
_____ External ear	_____ Round window	_____ Vestibulocochlear nerve

Record your observations for each of the following activities:

Rinne test: _____

_____

Weber test: _____

_____

Auditory acuity: _____

_____

Sound localization test: _____

_____

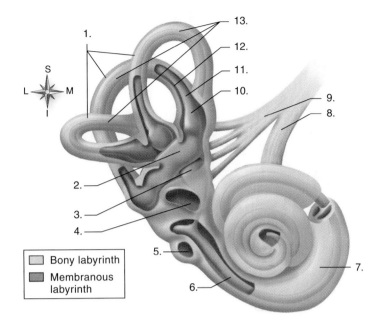

Figure 10.9

Relevant Terms			
_____	Ampulla	_____	Round window
_____	Cochlea	_____	Saccule (in vestibule)
_____	Cochlear duct	_____	Semicircular canals
_____	Cochlear nerve	_____	Semicircular ducts
_____	Endolymphatic space (within membrane)	_____	Utricle (in vestibule)
_____	Oval window	_____	Vestibular nerve
_____	Perilymphatic space		

Section C. Activities for the Gustatory and Olfactory Systems

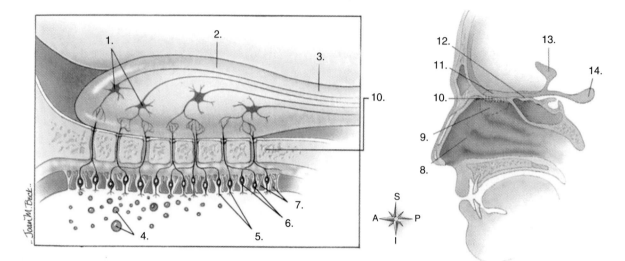

Figure 10.11

Relevant Terms	
_____ Cribriform plate (lamina cribrosa)	_____ Olfactory cilia
_____ Epithelial cells	_____ Olfactory epithelium
_____ Nasal cavity	_____ Olfactory nerves
_____ Olfactory bulb	_____ Olfactory tract
_____ Olfactory bulb	_____ Olfactory tract
_____ Olfactory cells	_____ Thalamic center
_____ Olfactory center	

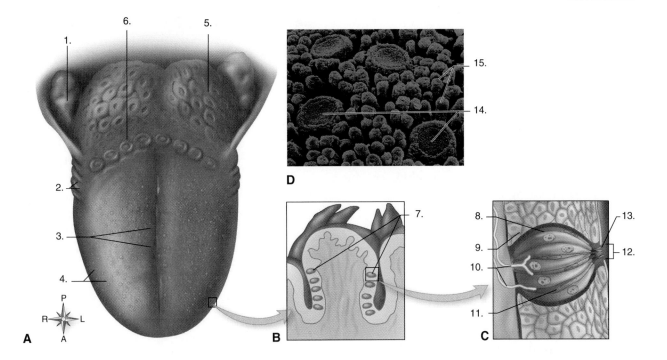

Figure 10.12

Relevant Terms	
_____ Circumvallate papillae	_____ Lingual tonsil
_____ Filiform papillae	_____ Nerve fibers
_____ Filiform papillae	_____ Oral epithelium
_____ Foliate papillae	_____ Palatine tonsil
_____ Fungiform papillae	_____ Supporting cell
_____ Fungiform papillae	_____ Taste buds
_____ Gustatory cell	_____ Taste pore
_____ Gustatory hairs	

Record your observations for each of the following activities:

Sense of smell:_____

_____

_____

Sense of taste: _____

_____

_____

Section B. Assessments

1. T/F The fluids in the eye help to focus incoming light.
2. T/F The bony labyrinth consists of the cochlea, the vestibule, and the tympanic membrane.
3. T/F Much of the sense of taste is actually affected by the sense of smell.
4. The organ primarily responsible for the sense of hearing is the:
   a. cochlea.
   b. organ of Corti.
   c. tympanic membrane.
   d. semicircular canal.
5. The sense of smell is due to the presence of:
   a. mechanoreceptors.
   b. proprioceptors.
   c. chemoreceptors.
   d. none of the above.
6. The "blind spot" of the eye is called the:
   a. optic disc.
   b. vitreous humor.
   c. fovea centralis.
   d. sclera.

Section C. Critical Thinking Problems

1. Research suggests that if the Snellen eye chart is reversed so that the largest font size is at the bottom, people read the smaller font size at the top more accurately than in a regular Snellen chart. It is conjectured that people's prior experience that the top lines on the chart are the easiest to read is responsible for improving their visual performance. How could this kind of conditioning be used to help people improve their vision? What are some ways that this could be used to hide information from people?

2. For most people, both vision and hearing are in 3D and with it comes greater sensory depth. While depth perception is an obvious benefit of stereoscopic vision, what advantages are there in stereophonic hearing? Is this a vital design component for an android?

Exercise 11

The Endocrine System

Overview

The human body is capable of adapting to a large number of environments, as evidenced by the various climates and extreme altitudes people can survive in, including the low orbit of the International Space Station. This is possible because of homeostasis, which involves the ability to dynamically adjust to changing conditions to establish a stable state. Machines also function in these environments, and must perform under various kinds of operating conditions. They may have controllers that regulate important internal systems, such as power usage, but these features are fundamentally different from the sophisticated control involved in homeostasis.

As AI researchers seek to develop androids, inevitably they will have to home in on mimicking the body's adaptability. This is a quite a challenge for an artificial system. Wherever people live, androids must be able to survive there too, whether in stable or dynamic environs. However, future artificial systems for homeostasis are ultimately achieved, they will have to communicate specifically to a multitude of components distributed throughout the android.

In the human body, homeostasis is accomplished by the nervous system in concert with a series of glands that secrete hormones as chemical "messengers" and are collectively known as the *endocrine system*. Through negative feedback loops, the endocrine system releases hormones to correct any deviations from the point of stability. In this exercise, we will explore the glands that make up the endocrine system.

Activity #1 — Endocrine Glands and Hormones

Introduction

The endocrine system, a handful of ductless glands distributed throughout the body, secretes hormones. These hormones have widespread influence once they circulate through the cardiovascular system and interact with specific cells. While the nervous system provides rapid communication to the body through electrical signals, the endocrine system operates at a much slower rate due to the diffusion of hormones from the ductless glands, through the bloodstream, and to their target cells. Despite the pace, the level of control is extremely precise because hormones only interact with certain cells. The release of a hormone is like a broadcast message to the body, but only the cells tuned into a particular frequency receive the message.

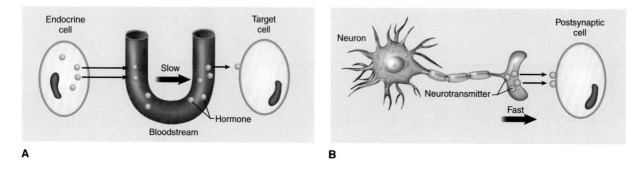

Figure 11.1 *Mechanisms of endocrine (A) and nervous (B) signals.*

Materials

Microscope
Microscope slides of the adrenal gland, the pancreas, and the thymus

---

Procedure

1. Review the section in your textbook related to the endocrine glands and hormones.
2. Endocrine glands are widely distributed and are often part of other organ systems. Identify the endocrine glands in Figure 11.2 in the Lab Report.
   a. The pea-sized pituitary gland, located on the interior of the brain off the hypothalamus, consists of two glands and releases a number of major hormones.
   b. The thyroid is a gland located just below the larynx on the surface of the trachea and regulates the metabolic rate of cells.
   c. Beneath the sternum, the thymus releases thymosin, which helps to regulate important immune cells (T cells).
   d. The adrenal glands, which sit on top of the kidneys, release hormones that regulate stress, especially cortisol and adrenaline.
   e. The pancreas is an exocrine and endocrine gland that releases insulin, produced by beta cells, which promotes the uptake of glucose into cells.
3. Examine Figure 11.3 of slides of tissue extracted from the adrenal gland, the pancreas, and the thymus. Use the figure to identify key structures in your own slides.

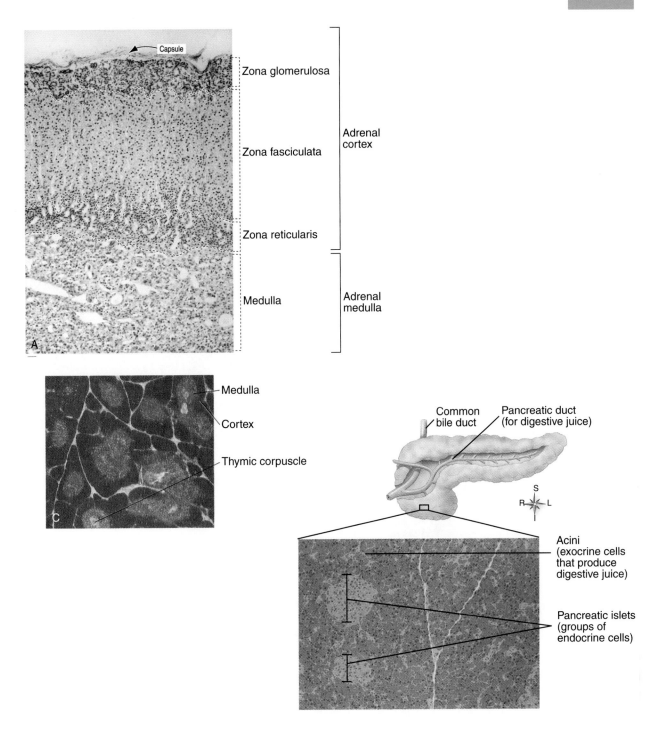

Capsule

Zona glomerulosa

Zona fasciculata — Adrenal cortex

Zona reticularis

Medulla — Adrenal medulla

A

Medulla

Cortex

Thymic corpuscle

C

Common bile duct

Pancreatic duct (for digestive juice)

S
R —✳— L

Acini (exocrine cells that produce digestive juice)

Pancreatic islets (groups of endocrine cells)

Figure 11.3

Lab Report for 11.1

Section A. Activities for the Endocrine Glands and Hormones

Figure 11.2

Relevant Terms	
_____ Adrenals	_____ Pineal
_____ Hypothalamus	_____ Pituitary
_____ Ovaries (female)	_____ Testes (male)
_____ Pancreas (islets)	_____ Thymus
_____ Parathyroids	_____ Thyroid

Record your observations.

Adrenal: _____

_____

_____

Pancreatic: _____

_____

_____

Thymic: _____

_____

_____

Section B. Assessments

1. T/F   The pancreas is both an endocrine and exocrine gland.
2. T/F   The function of the endocrine system is to regulate through chemical communication.
3. Beta cells in the pancreas are responsible for producing:
   a. cortisol.
   b. insulin.
   c. estrogen.
   d. human growth hormone.
4. The thymus gland:
   a. is located beneath the sternum.
   b. is important in the development of T cells.
   c. produces thymosin.
   d. all of the above.

Section C. Critical Thinking Problem

1. Considering the chemical structures of hormones, what can you speculate about the structure of the cellular receptors that are specific to a single hormone? (HINT: think of the lock-and-key mechanism for enzymes.)

Unit 4

Transportation and Defense

We make war that we may live in peace.

Aristotle

How does the body defend itself against foreign invasion?

The world is a dangerous place, but thanks to human ingenuity, strategies and technological improvements have been developed that have resulted in the doubling of human life expectancy since the 18th century. Yet one of the greatest daily threats to an individual's health remains the ceaseless barrage of pathogens against the body's defenses.

Though the unaided human eye cannot directly witness this fight, the battle against viruses, bacteria, and other microorganisms is ongoing and intense. In fact, at the microscopic level, life can be better defined in terms of waging war.

Despite all the attacks, the body overwhelmingly achieves victory over pathogens. This is possible because of the solid defense of its territorial borders, defined by the integumentary system. When pathogens do make it past the border, lymph draws them into the lymph nodes, which serve as garrisons for the immune cell forces. And just as wars are often won or lost over supply lines, the body relies on both the cardiovascular and lymphatic systems for vital transport to keep its troops supplied, connected, and mobile.

To appreciate this cellular theater of war, this unit will relate features of the cardiovascular, lymphatic, immune, and integumentary systems to analogous counterparts in a military force tasked with defending its homeland.

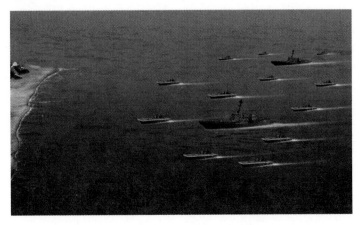

217

Exercise 12
The Cardiovascular System

Lesson Overview

Activity #1: Blood
  Part A: Composition
  Part B: Blood Types
Activity #2: Blood Vessels and the Paths of Circulation
Activity #3: The Heart
  Part A: Anatomy of the Heart
  Part B: The Cardiac Cycle and Vital Signs
Evolve Activity #1: WBC and RBC Counts
Evolve Activity #2: Hematocrit
Evolve Activity #3: Electrocardiography

Overview

At the heart of every great military is a rapid and reliable transportation system enabling both troops and resources to move uninhibited. Part of the success of the ancient Roman Empire was the extensive system of roads that radiated out from Rome used for transportation and communication, which inspired the saying, "All roads lead to Rome." Today, the U.S. military utilizes 61,000 miles of highways across the United States to move personnel and equipment as part of its Strategic Highway Network, which is vital to the support of military forces and the defense of its borders.

In the human body, resources and defense forces are transported through a closed network called the *circulatory system*, comprised of the cardiovascular system, including the heart and blood vessels for the movement of blood, and the lymphatic system, which is a series of ducts connected by lymphatic vessels, that transports lymph.

In this exercise, we focus on the cardiovascular system, beginning with a detailed look at blood, followed by an examination of the heart, and finally the cardiovascular pathway; that is, the two separate circuits through which blood flows throughout the body.

Activity #1 — Blood

Part A: Composition of Blood

Introduction

Blood has been called the *currency of war*. In the war being waged against the body, blood is the support system, a means of transport for supplies in the form of nutrients, cellular defense forces, components that repair tissue, and a means for waste to be removed. Blood allows the front lines of the body to be patrolled and maintained continuously. Every organ in the body relies upon the nutrients delivered by blood.

Although popular depictions of the armed forces usually involve images of soldiers, a large number of personnel in the military serve in support roles, many of whom never see combat. A variety of business contractors and civilian employees also work in support roles for the military. The diverse combat and non-combat personnel must work alongside one another in times of peace and war as a single unit to defend a nation.

Similarly, blood carries over 100 different components, yet appears as a single substance to the human eye. It is a connective tissue consisting of an almost 1:1 ratio of various cells and platelets, called *formed elements*, suspended in a fluid matrix called *plasma*, which contains water, electrolytes, nutrients and variety of other components. The three types of formed elements are red blood cells (RBCs) or erythrocytes, white blood cells (WBCs) or leukocytes, and platelets. Analogous to a military force, leukocytes are the combat personnel, intelligence officers, spies, diplomats, strategists, and generals that serve their designated defense functions in the immune system. Erythrocytes are support cells transporting the vital resource, oxygen, and platelets perform maintenance functions, helping to repair damage to vessels through the formation of blood clots.

Materials

Microscope
Prepared microscope slides of human blood

Procedure

1. Review the section in your textbook related to the composition of blood.

Differential White Blood Cell Count

2. A differential white blood cell count is a useful test to identify the types of WBCs present in a blood sample. Note that the test doesn't tell you the total percent of WBCs in blood, but instead provides the distribution of the different types of WBCs present. This is useful in that abnormal percentages of leukocytes can indicate the presence of particular diseases.

3. WBCs are nucleated cells that appear stained (if the sample has been prepared with Wright stain) when viewed with a microscope. Many are larger than RBCs and have distinct features, allowing them to be identified according to Figure 12.2.

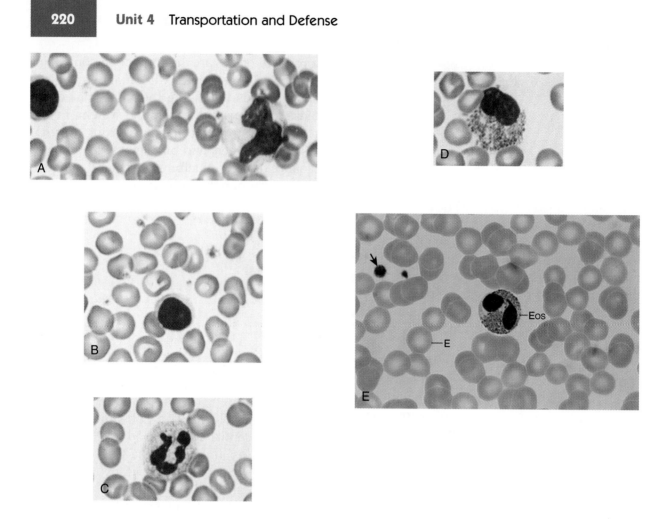

Figure 12.2 *Representative human blood cells.* **A**, *monocyte.* **B**, *lymphocyte.* **C**, *neutrophil.* **D**, *basophil.* **E**, *erythrocyte. (E, erythrocyte; Eos, eosinophil; arrow, platelet.)*

4. You will be counting 100 WBCs on the slide. Having a cover slide with a grid may be helpful for your counts. It is important that you move the slide so that you do not double count, so a common counting method is to slowly move the slide as shown in Figure 12.3.

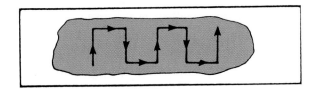

Figure 12.3

5. Record the numbers of each of the various types of WBCs present in your sample until you have identified 100 WBCs total. Add up the amount of each type of WBC and record it as a percentage present in the blood in your lab report.

Part B: Blood Types

Introduction

While militaries strive to operate as cohesive units, especially in the face of an enemy, internal conflicts can still arise. Competitiveness can occur between different branches of the armed services, such as during the annual Army/Navy football game, or even between enlisted and civilian personnel. This interservice rivalry can have a morale-boosting effect, building stronger connections and instilling greater loyalty among personnel within a particular branch. Taken too far, however, infighting can become detrimental.

On its own, blood within the human body functions effectively, just like a branch of the military working with its own people. However, a kind of interservice rivalry can occur when blood from two individuals is mixed, such as during a blood transfusion. If there is a mismatch in the blood types, problems arise due to a class of proteins within plasma known as *antibodies*. These proteins bind to specific antigen glycoproteins on the surface of RBCs that do not match the genetically determined RBCs in the body receiving the new blood. "Infighting" breaks out, and foreign RBCs clump together and are ruptured. Fortunately, blood types can be differentiated through ABO and Rh blood typing, which prevents detrimental transfusions from occurring.

Materials

Fresh blood sample or artificial blood samples for blood typing
Blood typing kit
Microscope slides
Wax pencil
Toothpicks

Before You Begin

- *Always wear latex gloves and protective eyewear when handling blood.*
- *To avoid blood clotting, work quickly once the blood has been exposed to air. If it's heparinized (commercial) you have more time — if not, you must collect it using heparinized blood collection capillary tubes.*

Procedure

1. Review the section in your textbook related to ABO and Rh blood types.

ABO System

2. The ABO system for blood typing is a visual test that allows for the rapid identification of A and B antigens present in a blood sample. Blood may contain both (type AB), one (type A or B), or none (type O) of the antigens. To determine whether antigens are present, blood is mixed with serum containing anti-A or anti-B antibodies, which will cause agglutination if the matching corresponding antigen is present.

3. On a clean microscope slide, divide the slide into two halves using a wax pencil labeling the left half "anti-A" and the right half "anti-B."

4. Add a drop of the anti-A serum to blood in the left half and a drop of the anti-B serum to the blood on the right half.

5. Place a small drop of blood in each half. Using separate toothpicks, stir the blood and serum in each half together and spread the mixture out into a larger circle, but not so thin that it will dry rapidly.

6. After 2 minutes, examine both samples for the presence of clumping (not clotting), using Figure 12.4 (below) to aid you:

Rh System

7. The Rh system for blood typing identifies the common Rh or D antigen. The clumping is not as distinct as in ABO typing, so clumps will be smaller, making them more difficult to observe.

8. On a clean microscope slide, add a drop of anti-D serum.

9. Place a small drop of blood onto the serum droplet and place the slide on a slide warmer that is prewarmed to 45° C. The slide warmer will tilt the slide back and forth to encourage the antigen-antibody reaction. In some cases, it may not be necessary to heat the slide.

10. At 2 minutes, assess whether the sample contains any clumping. If clumping occurred within 2 minutes, the blood type is Rh positive, otherwise it is Rh negative.

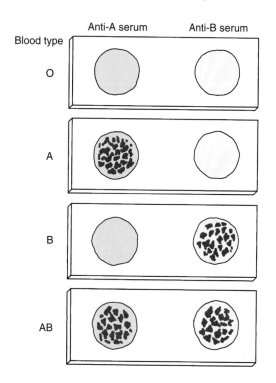

Figure 12.4

Lab Report for 12.1

Section A. Activities for Blood

Differential WBC Count Tally Grid					
Type	**Monocyte**	**Lymphocyte**	**Neutrophil**	**Eosinophil**	**Basophil**
Tally marks:					
Totals:					
Percentages:					

Key: Percentage = (number observed / total counted or 100) X 100

Section B. Activities for Blood Types

Blood Test Results			
Subject:			Sex: ❑ male ❑ female
Test	**Normal Value**	**Result**	**Interpretation**
WBC count			
RBC count			
Hematocrit			
Hemoglobin			
Method: _____			
ABO type			

Section C. Assessments

1. T/F Plasma consists of mostly of water.
2. T/F An individual with both A and B antigens on his red blood cells but lacking antibodies in the plasma would have type O blood.
3. T/F The Rh factor is part of the blood plasma.
4. Plasma consists of:
   a. waste products from metabolism.
   b. digested food.
   c. proteins.
   d. all of the above.

5. Approximately how many red blood cells are in a cubic millimeter of blood?
   a. 50,000
   b. 500,000
   c. 5,000,000
   d. 50,000,000
6. Red blood cells are also known as:
   a. erythrocytes.
   b. eosinophils.
   c. leukocytes.
   d. thrombocytes.

7. A blood sample with antigen A on blood cells and anti-B antibody in the plasma is type:
   a. O.
   b. AB.
   c. A.
   d. B.

2. It is still somewhat of a mystery why there are different blood types. From an evolutionary point of view, what possible advantages or disadvantages would the presence of different blood types contribute to the welfare of the human race as a whole?

Section D. Critical Thinking Problems

1. For all the advertisements about keeping various parts of the body healthy, including skin, hair, teeth, and bones, little attention is given to blood health. Some aspects are addressed in public awareness pamphlets or posters about blood-borne or sexually transmitted disease, but rarely is the subject of blood health addressed directly. What issues could be addressed to help the public improve blood health?

Activity #2 — Blood Vessels and the Paths of Circulation

Introduction

Regardless of sheer military might, if an army cannot get to the front lines in an effective and orderly manner, it is powerless. This underscores the importance of training and planning for deployment. Furthermore, the best militaries constantly review their current procedures to ensure efficient mobilization, revising strategic routes based on needs; changing meteorological, sociological, and political conditions; and even new technology. Military history has many examples of victory over an enemy simply through better organization in the deployment of troops and supplies.

Cardiovascular pathways are the body's means of deploying vital components to tissues. These pathways consist of a network of interconnected vessels divided into two paths: the pulmonary loop (cycling blood from the heart to the lungs and back) and the systemic loop (cycling blood from the heart to the rest of the body and back). The pathways contain various-sized blood vessels with the smallest being capillaries. In the systemic loop, oxygenated blood is transported away from the heart through arteries and deoxygenated blood returns to the heart through veins. In the pulmonary loop, deoxygenated blood flows through arteries to the lungs to become oxygenated and returns to the heart through the pulmonary veins.

Materials

Human body models, heart models, posters, and dissections (head, torso, limbs) showing cardiovascular pathways

Procedure

1. Review the section in your textbook related to blood vessels and cardiovascular paths.
2. Examine the diagram in Figure 12.5 of blood vessels and identify the major structures, including the three major tunics of vessels.
3. Identify the major arteries of the body according to Figure 12.6 (you may also use models to help you, if available).
4. Identify the major veins of the body according to Figure 12.7 (you may also use models to help you, if available).
5. The hepatic portal system is a venous portion of the systemic loop that delivers blood from the intestine to the liver in order to process absorbed substances before reaching the heart. Of note, blood in the hepatic portal travels from a capillary bed to another capillary bed before heading back to the heart. Use Figure 12.8 to identify the important vessels in this system.

Lab Report for 12.2

Section A. Activities for Blood Vessels and the Paths of Circulation

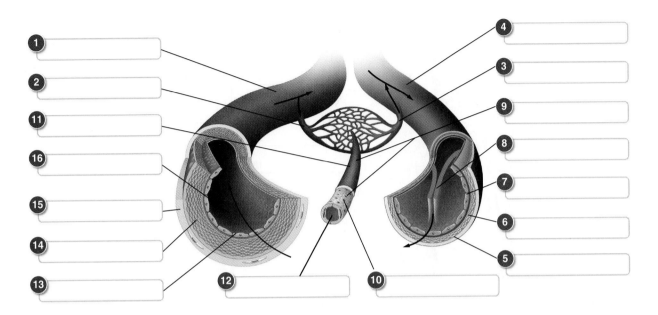

Figure 12.5

Relevant Terms	
Arteriole	Tunica intima
Artery	Tunica intima
Capillary	Tunica intima
Endothelium	Tunica media
Loose connective tissue	Tunica media
Lumen	Valve
Tunica externa	Vein
Tunica externa	Venule

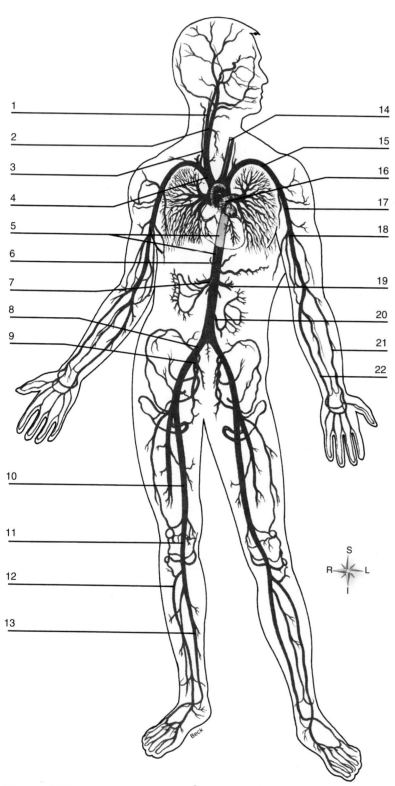

Relevant Terms
_____ Anterior tibial
_____ Aorta
_____ Axillary
_____ Brachial
_____ Brachiocephalic
_____ Celiac
_____ Common iliac
_____ External carotid
_____ Femoral
_____ Inferior mesenteric
_____ Internal carotid
_____ Internal iliac
_____ Left common carotid
_____ Popliteal
_____ Posterior tibial
_____ Pulmonary
_____ Radial
_____ Renal
_____ Right common carotid
_____ Subclavian
_____ Superior mesenteric
_____ Ulnar

Figure 12.6

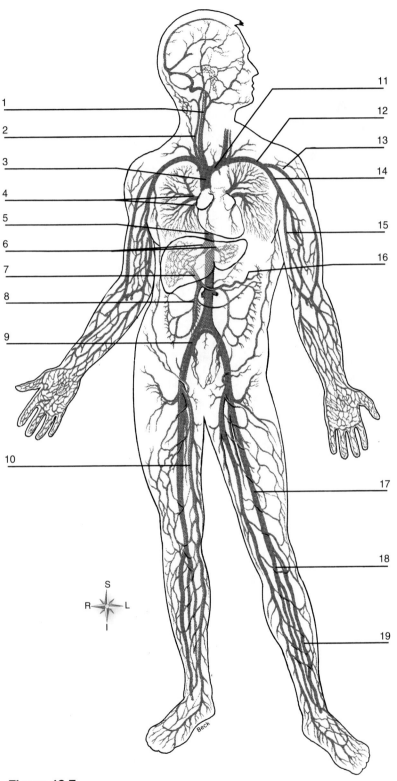

Relevant Terms
_____ Anterior tibial
_____ Axillary
_____ Basilic
_____ Cephalic
_____ Common iliac
_____ External jugular
_____ Femoral
_____ Great saphenous
_____ Hepatic
_____ Hepatic portal
_____ Inferior vena cava
_____ Internal jugular
_____ Left brachiocephalic
_____ Popliteal
_____ Pulmonary
_____ Splenic
_____ Subclavian
_____ Superior mesenteric
_____ Superior vena cava

Figure 12.7

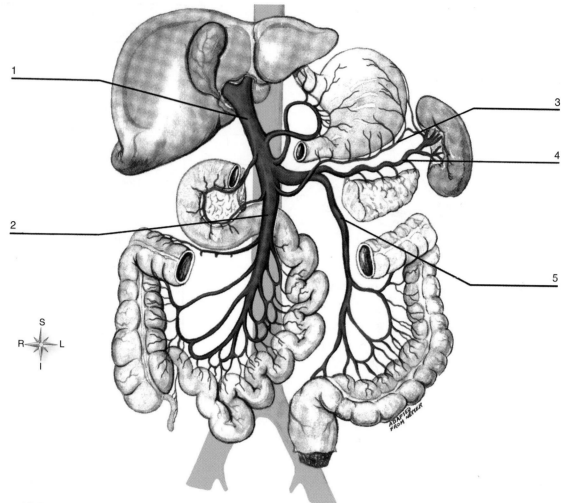

Figure 12.8

Relevant Terms
_____ Gastroepiploic
_____ Hepatic portal
_____ Inferior mesenteric
_____ Splenic
_____ Superior mesenteric

Section B. Assessments

1. T/F   Arteries always carry blood to the heart.
2. T/F   Pulmonary circulation begins in the left ventricle or aorta and ends in the vena cava or right atrium.
3. T/F   Blood leaving the liver connects to the inferior vena cava through the hepatic portal vein.
4. The last blood vessel in the pulmonary circulation circuit is the:
   a. superior vena cava.
   b. pulmonary vein.
   c. pulmonary artery.
   d. aorta.
5. Smooth muscle tissue is located in which layer of the arteries and veins?
   a. tunica media
   b. tunica intima
   c. endothelium
   d. none of the above

Section C. Critical Thinking Problem

1. Although at first glance cardiovascular pathways seem complex, they are far less complicated than other networks. They are simplified because they are driven by a single pump (the heart) and the paths are cyclic. The systemic pathway is the larger loop and the pulmonary loop a simpler and shorter circuit. But what if the anatomy was different? Consider the following possibilities and list a benefit and detriment for each:
   a. Two hearts in the cardiovascular system

   b. Paths that are not cyclic/closed

   c. Two or more major pathways

Activity #3 — The Heart

Part A: Anatomy of the Heart

Introduction

Militaries are known for extensive organizational structure, sometimes to a fault. Between the heads of the military to the lowest soldiers, numerous branches, departments, sections, and other divisions have been devised and arranged into a hierarchy that can be quite complex. Yet these groupings are necessary for the delegation of tasks and ensuring order and accountability within the ranks. The entire military depends on each department working correctly in order to function in an ever-ready state.

In a related way, the heart is an organ divided into chambers that work in succession, ensuring that blood flows continually throughout the body. Each step in the sequence is vital in order for the heart to beat billions of times in the course of an average human lifespan. The function of each chamber and its role in the cardiac cycle will be investigated in the next activity; but first, an understanding of the anatomy of the heart is necessary to grasp all that occurs in a single heartbeat.

Materials

Model of the heart
Preserved mammalian heart, such as a sheep's heart
Stethoscopes
Sphygmomanometers

Procedure

1. Review the section in your textbook related to the anatomy of the heart.
2. Examine the model and Figure 12.9 in the Lab Report to identify the heart's surface features.
3. Examine the internal anatomy of the heart to identify the key structures in Figure 12.10 in the Lab Report.

Part B: The Cardiac Cycle and Vital Signs

Introduction

The heart is the driving force within the cardiovascular system. It is a biological pump in which chemical energy is used to create pressure in the blood to push it through the system. The cardiac cycle of the heart involves a systematic sequence that regulates pumping action, timed to ensure repeatability as well as flexibility in its pumping rate. Because of the closed nature of the cardiovascular system, blood flow is defined along well-constructed pathways, much like roads and transport routes define the paths of troop transport for military forces.

The overall function of the heart is to cycle oxygenated and deoxygenated blood through proper circuits. In carrying out this function, the heart goes through a sequence of actions called the *cardiac cycle*. Pumping of the ventricles and atria is regulated by signals from the brain through sympathetic nerves and spontaneous depolarizations from cells in the sinoatrial (SA) node, located in the right atrium. Collectively, these cells act as a biological pacemaker to reset the cardiac cycle. Other cells in the atrioventricular (AV) junction and the ventricles can fire independently of nerve impulses, albeit at lower rates. In other words, while the brain plays a role in controlling the heart rate, cells in the heart can operate independently for short periods of time.

Much of the cardiac cycle can be ascertained without ever seeing the heart directly, as you will observe in the following activity.

> **Materials**
>
> Model of the heart
> Preserved mammalian heart, such as a sheep's
> or cow's heart

Procedure

1. Review the section in your textbook related to the anatomy of the heart.

The Radial Pulse

2. When blood is pumped through vessels, the pressure caused by each ventricular contraction causes the vessel to swell temporarily, and then recoil as the pressure subsides. The force exerted by the heart on the blood translates into this "pulse" of the vessels, which can be felt throughout the body.

3. Taking a pulse involves a simple palpitation with your fingers. A radial pulse can be easily taken by applying pressure with two fingers (but not the thumb) on the anterior surface of the wrist, which may push an artery against the radius allowing you to detect the pulses in the vessel.

4. Count the number of pulses you feel in 15 seconds and multiply this number by 4 to obtain the pulse rate per minute.

5. If a pulse cannot be obtained on the wrist, try other locations shown in Figure 12.11:

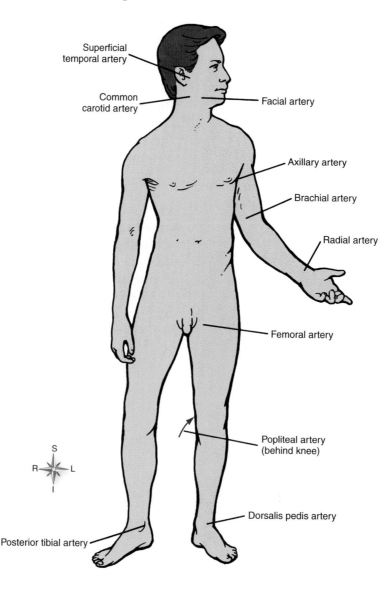

Figure 12.11

Heart Sounds and the Apical Pulse

6. The pumping of the heart can be detected audibly with a stethoscope, allowing for rapid assessment of heart activity. The pumping sequence is a three-step pattern commonly called *lub-dup-pause*. The louder "lub" sound corresponds to the closing of the AV valves, which occurs during systole or ventricular contraction. The "dup" sound occurs during diastole or ventricular relaxation and is the sound of the semilunar (SL) valves closing.

7. To hear the heart pumping, obtain a stethoscope and clean the earpieces with alcohol swabs. Place the earpieces in your ears and rotate them about 15 degrees forward toward the bridge of your nose for comfort.

8. Place the diaphragm or bell of the stethoscope on a subject's (or your) exposed chest, approximately near the apex of the heart at the fifth intercostal space. Listen carefully for the pumping sequence described above and describe it, making sure to identify the lub and dup portions. Attempt to time the length of the pause in the pumping sequence.

9. Breathe deeply a few times and time the pause in the pumping sequence.

10. Do some simple exercises, such as push-ups, jumping jacks, or running in place for 1 minute, and time the pause in the pumping sequence.

11. To take an apical pulse, simply count the number of pulses you hear in 15 seconds and multiply this number by 4 to obtain the pulse rate per minute.

Blood Pressure

12. The subject whose blood pressure will be monitored should be relaxed in an upright position. The most common location to take the blood pressure is to monitor the brachial artery at the antecubital space. Wrap the cuff of the sphygmomanometer about an inch above the bend of the elbow with the inflatable bladder on the medial surface of the arm. Make sure it is snug but not uncomfortable. Use Figure 12.12 to aid in the procedure.

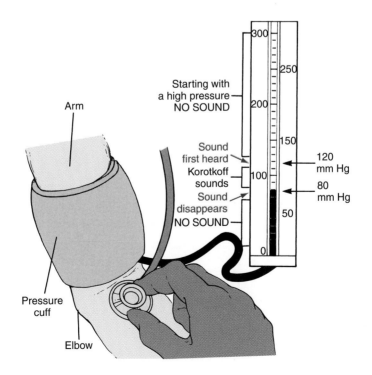

Figure 12.12

13. Place the stethoscope diaphragm on the brachial artery under the cuff and just medial to the bend of the elbow. Close the valve on the sphygmomanometer bulb. While palpating the radial pulse and watching the gauge on the sphygmomanometer, inflate the cuff (or have someone else inflate the cuff if you are taking your own blood pressure) to around 150 mm Hg or about 30 mm Hg above when you can no longer feel a pulse. At this point, the vessel will be occluded so work fast — do not keep the pressure on this vessel for longer than absolutely necessary.

14. Slowly open the bulb valve to release pressure at a rate of about 2-3 mm Hg per second. Listen for Korotkoff sounds, which are loud tapping noises in the artery, and record the pressure when they begin. This pressure is the systolic pressure, which is high enough to briefly open the vessel.

15. Continue to decrease the pressure until the Korotkoff sounds dissipate and the blood flows freely in the artery. Record the pressure when the sounds can no longer be heard; this is the diastolic pressure. At this point, even the lowest pressure in the vessel is enough to keep it open.

16. Open the valve all the way and release the pressure from the bulb.

17. Repeat the above procedure a few times to obtain an average blood pressure reading, which is expressed as the systolic pressure over the diastolic pressure with the average pressure being "120 over 80." Do not do more than three measurements on one arm.

18. Have the subject (which may be you) exercise for 3 minutes and then immediately take a blood pressure measurement.

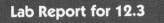

Lab Report for 12.3

Section A. Activities for the Heart

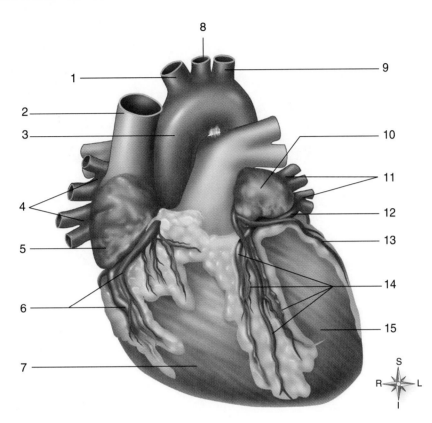

Figure 12.9

Relevant Terms	
_____ Anterior interventricular branches of left coronary artery and cardiac vein	_____ Left subclavian artery
_____ Ascending aorta	_____ Left ventricle
_____ Brachiocephalic trunk	_____ Right atrium
_____ Circumflex artery	_____ Right coronary artery and cardiac vein
_____ Great cardiac vein	_____ Right pulmonary veins
_____ Left atrium	_____ Right ventricle
_____ Left common carotid artery	_____ Superior vena cava
_____ Left pulmonary veins	

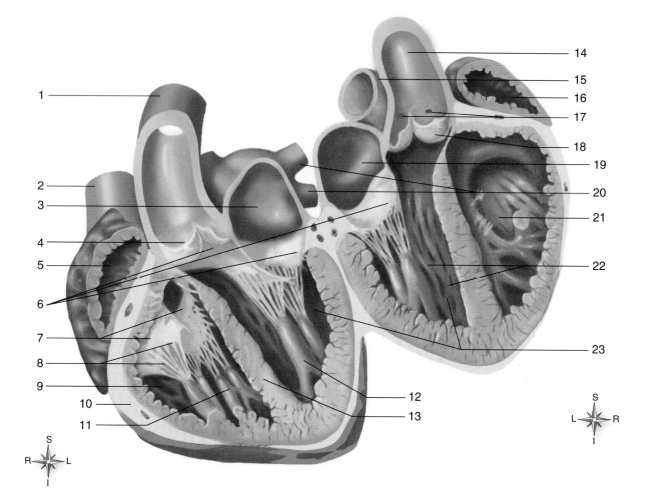

Figure 12.10

Relevant Terms		
_____ Aorta	_____ Left atrium	_____ Right atrium
_____ Aorta	_____ Left AV (mitral) valve	_____ Right atrium
_____ Aortic (SL) valve	_____ Left ventricle	_____ Right AV (tricuspid) valve
_____ Aortic (SL) valve	_____ Openings to coronary arteries	_____ Right ventricle
_____ Chordae tendineae	_____ Papillary muscle	_____ Right ventricle
_____ Fatty connective tissue	_____ Papillary muscle	_____ Superior vena cava
_____ Interventricular septum	_____ Pulmonary trunk	_____ Trabeculae carneae
_____ Left atrium	_____ Pulmonary veins	

Section B. Activities for the Cardiac Cycle and Vital Signs

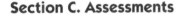

Section C. Assessments

1. T/F The apex of the heart is its blunted point.
2. T/F The pacemaker of the heart is the sinoatrial node.
3. T/F Valves ensure that blood flow in the heart goes in both directions.
4. The first heart sound that can be heard in the cardiac cycle is the closing of the:
   a. mitral and bicuspid valves.
   b. tricuspid and mitral valves.
   c. tricuspid and pulmonary semilunar valves.
   d. pulmonary semilunar and aortic semilunar valves.
5. The upper chambers of the heart:
   a. discharge blood.
   b. are called *ventricles*.
   c. receive blood.
   d. both a and b above.
6. Which of the following is true about the pulse?
   a. A pulse cannot be taken in the lower body.
   b. It must be taken with veins.
   c. It can only be felt in arteries.
   d. Only a vein passing over a bone provides a reliable pulse.

Section D. Critical Thinking Problem

1. The cardiovascular system is a closed circuit involving separate networks of tubes connected to two pumps integrated into one device so that the fluid within can be effectively recycled through the entire system.

   While this explanation may sound like it is from a technical handbook, the reality is that the cardiovascular system is a highly complicated system to study, so much so that an international journal called *Cardiovascular Engineering* exists to address the application of engineering concepts to its study and health. In general, engineers utilize scientific principles to solve practical problems. What aspects of the cardiovascular system would benefit from an engineer's point of view?

Exercise 13

The Lymphatic and Immune Systems

Lesson Overview

Activity #1: Nodes, Organs, and Pathways in the Lymphatic System

Activity #2: The Immune Response

Overview

Militaries are often responsible for carrying out more than just the preparations for and execution of battle. Armed forces cooperate with local officials to assist in peacekeeping efforts, including providing food and supplies, maintaining roads, and making areas habitable after natural disasters. Of course, this is not purely for humanitarian purposes; it is a significant part of military strategy. After all, instability in a region due to poor living conditions or the lack of vital resources can lead to civil unrest or be capitalized upon by enemies.

In this regard, the lymphatic system resembles the supporting role of the military. Not only does the lymphatic system aid in the production and transport of cellular forces that are part of the immune system, it also plays a role in the digestion of absorbed substances from the digestive tract, and maintains proper extracellular fluid balance by removing excess fluid. With its network of vessels, as extensive as those of the cardiovascular system, the lymphatic system serves as a multifunctional line of defense in the body.

In this exercise, we will first examine lymph nodes and lymphatic pathways, and then turn our attention to the immune response.

Activity #1 — Nodes, Organs, and Pathways in the Lymphatic System

Introduction

The U.S. Department of Defense manages approximately half a million buildings at more than 5,000 sites worldwide. These facilities, used to house and train personnel and store equipment, are strategically located to enable operations in times of peace and war.

Lymph nodes, or glands, and lymphatic organs serve as garrisons for cells of the immune system and are linked through an elaborate network of pathways. Hundreds of lymph nodes are grouped into strategic clusters throughout the body. As lymph flows through the system, materials or microorganisms carried from tissues trigger nodes into action, both in the production of lymphocytes and in the destruction of invaders.

Immune cells may be the soldiers in the battle to defend against invaders, but it is the nodes and organs of the lymphatic system that serve as localized theaters of operation for warfare against the body's enemies.

Materials

Model of the torso and head
Model of the lymphatic system, if available
Microscope
Histological slides of the tonsil, spleen and thymus

Procedure

1. Review the section in your textbook related to the lymphatic nodes and vessels.
2. Identify the key structures of a lymph node in Figure 13.1 in the Lab Report.
3. Examine Figure 13.2 in the Lab Report, which shows the lymphatic system, and identify the key lymph organs and nodes.
4. Examine each of the slides and sketch what you observe. Be sure to identify the structures found in Figure 13.3 in the Lab Report.

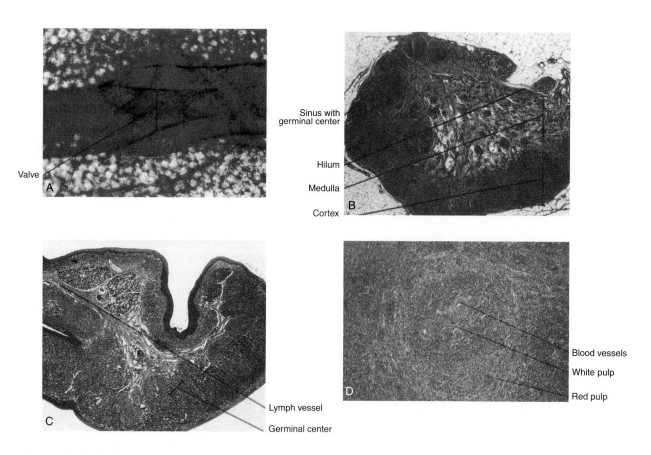

Figure 13.3 **A**, *lymphatic vessel.* **B**, *lymph node.* **C**, *palatine tonsil.* **D**, *spleen tissue.*

Lab Report for 13.1

Section A. Activities for Nodes, Organs, and Pathways in the Lymphatic System

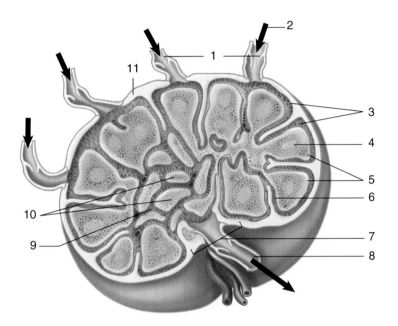

Figure 13.1

Relevant Terms			
_____	Afferent lymph vessels	_____	Lymph
_____	Capsule	_____	Medullary cords
_____	Cortical nodules	_____	Medullary sinus
_____	Efferent lymph vessel	_____	Sinuses
_____	Germinal center	_____	Trabeculae
_____	Hilum		

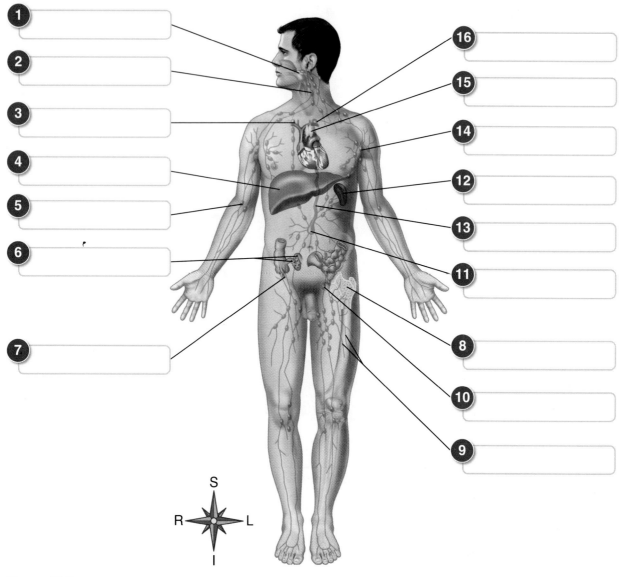

1

2

3

4

5

6

7

16

15

14

12

13

11

8

10

9

S

R — L

I

Figure 13.2

Relevant Terms	
Aggregated lymphoid nodules (Peyer patches)	Lymphatic vessels
Appendix	Red bone marrow
Axillary lymph node	Right lymphatic duct
Cervical lymph node	Spleen
Cisterna chyli	Superficial cubital (supratrochlear lymph nodes
Entrance of thoracic duct into subclavian vein	Thoracic duct
Inguinal lymph node	Thymus gland
Liver	Tonsils

Tonsil

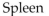

Spleen

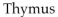

Thymus

Section B. Assessments

1. T/F Lymph nodes are unable to filter bacteria from lymph.
2. T/F Lymph is carried away from lymph nodes by efferent vessels.
3. T/F One-way valves in lymph vessels ensure that lymph flows in only one direction.
4. Which of the following structures is NOT part of the lymphatic system?
   a. appendix
   b. thymus
   c. spleen
   d. kidney

5. Which of the following is NOT a structure within a lymph node?
   a. nodule
   b. gray matter
   c. hilum
   d. capsule

Section C. Critical Thinking Problem

1. Imagine you were the body's general of the immune system and it was up to you to map out the locations of the lymph nodes and lymphatic organs in the body. Would you select the same locations for the clusters found in the body, namely the groin, armpits, and neck? Explain your answer.

Activity #2 — Immune Response

Introduction

Some enemies opt to remain hidden, waiting for an opportune moment to attack. When it comes to the global stage, it is often difficult for one nation to identify its enemies versus its allies, especially in the modern age. Modern militaries must have one foot in diplomacy and the other in intelligence in order to identify adversarial persons, groups, or nations. Once an enemy is discovered, it is in the nation's best interest to take the proper course of action, be it violent or nonviolent, in order to reduce the threat to its well-being.

The process that the body uses to identify and deal with an enemy is known as an *immune response* and it plays out at the molecular level. An immune response occurs when components of the immune system recognize foreign invaders — whether substances, viruses, or bacteria — and take action to defend the body against them. Immune system components are on patrol seeking out antigens, typically proteins that lie on the surface of various pathogens, although they can also be drugs, toxins, foreign material, and other chemicals. Antigens are detected when they bind to specific antibodies that are either attached to the surface of lymphocytes or are free after being released by them. Once bound, a sequence of events is initiated in order to destroy the foreign invaders rapidly.

In order to appreciate the importance of the mechanism behind how the body identifies its enemy, a closer look at antigen recognition through antibody binding is warranted.

Materials

Bio-Rad's ELISA Immuno Explorer™ kit
Micropipets
Micropipet tips
Buffer solution
Paper towels

Procedure

1. Review immune cells in section 4.1 of this manual and the immune response in your textbook.
2. An enzyme-linked immunosorbent assay, or ELISA, is a diagnostic technique to detect the presence of antigens in a sample. The way this is done is analogous to what occurs in the body when antibodies bind to foreign antigens. In the assay, a specific antibody bound to an enzyme will produce a color change in a solution when the corresponding antigen is present in the sample, while no color change will be produced if the antigen is not present. This provides a convenient and rapid test to detect specific antigens. While ELISA technology has been used in a variety of functions, including pregnancy and drug tests, you will be using the kit to simulate the detection of pathogenic antigens by antibodies.
3. Workstations set up by your instructor will provide all the materials you need to complete the lab.
4. Be sure to record all of your findings in the space provided in your lab report.

Lab Report for 13.2

Section A. Activities for Immune Cells and Response

Record your observations and results of the ELISA test:

_____

_____

_____

_____

_____

_____

_____

_____

Section B. Assessments

1. T/F   An antibody and an antigen fit together like a key in a lock.
2. T/F   A protein on the surface of a microorganism or cancer cell can be an antigen.
3. Antibodies are produced by:
   a. neutrophils.
   b. lymphocytes.
   c. macrophages.
   d. none of the above.

Section C. Critical Thinking Problem

1. Every human cell also has antigens on its surface. What is the point of these antigens and what possible complications can occur with the immune system because of their existence?

Exercise 14
The Integumentary System

Overview

In military terminology, the forward-most position of combat forces in a conflict is called the *front line*. It serves as the first defense against any hostile forces and can include a variety of different weapons, structures or personnel. Unlike a physical barrier, such as the Great Wall of China, a military front line is a dynamic entity, even when maintaining a relatively static position.

In terms of the body's ability to defend itself against foreign invasion, the integumentary system serves as the front line, a dynamic structure consisting of many components within the skin. It is the largest organ in the body, serving as a protective cover for tissues underneath it as well as disposing of foreign contaminants or pathogens through the routine shedding of skin cells.

In this exercise, we will take a brief look at the structure of the skin in order to appreciate its complexity.

Activity #1 — Structure of the Skin

Introduction

Our skin may be the most memorable aspect of who we are. Consider how much we can assess about someone based on his or her skin. It is a primary feature in the facial recognition that occurs in the brain. It reveals hidden details about hygiene and radiates touches of beauty. It serves as a record of accidents through scars and is a canvas for birthmarks, freckles, moles, and other colorations. It is both a window into the past, as wrinkles reveal a person's age or sun exposure, and a diagnostic tool of the present, such as whether someone is flushed. It even serves as a location of disease, such as skin cancer. More than ever, we are concerned about both the health and aesthetics of our skin.

Though soldiers are sent to fight in extreme conditions, they are still expected to present with flawless service uniforms. Militaries are incredibly concerned about how they are perceived outwardly as a sign of how they work internally and of their ability to fight an enemy.

In this activity, you will study the anatomy of the skin to appreciate to gain a better sense of this organ of defense.

Materials
Microscope
Histological slides of the skin

Procedure

1. Review the section in your textbook related to the integumentary system.
2. Identify the key structures of skin in Figure 14.1.
3. Identify the key structures in the histological slides of skin tissue in Figure 14.2.
4. Examine the slides of skin tissue provided by your instructor. Use the space in the lab report to sketch what you observe.

Lab Report for 14.1

Section A. Activities for the Structure of the Skin

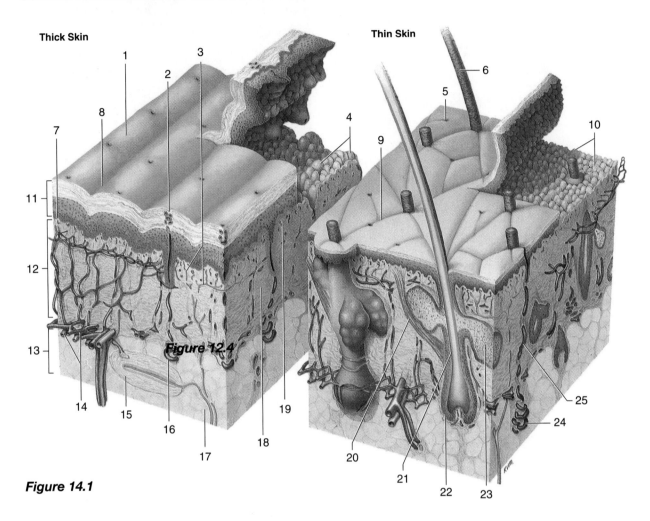

Figure 14.1

Relevant Terms		
Thick Skin		**Thin Skin**
_____ Blood vessels	_____ Papillary layer of dermis	_____ Sweat gland
_____ Dermis	_____ Reticular layer of dermis	_____ Arrector pili muscle
_____ Dermo-epidermal junction	_____ Ridges of dermal papillae	_____ Dermal papillae
_____ Epidermis	_____ Subcutaneous adipose tissue	_____ Hair follicle
_____ Friction ridge	_____ Sulcus	_____ Hair shaft
_____ Hypodermis	_____ Sweat duct	_____ Opening of sweat duct
_____ Lamellar (Pacini) corpuscle	_____ Sweat gland	_____ Root of hair
_____ Nerve fibers		_____ Sebaceous gland
		_____ Sulcus
		_____ Sweat duct

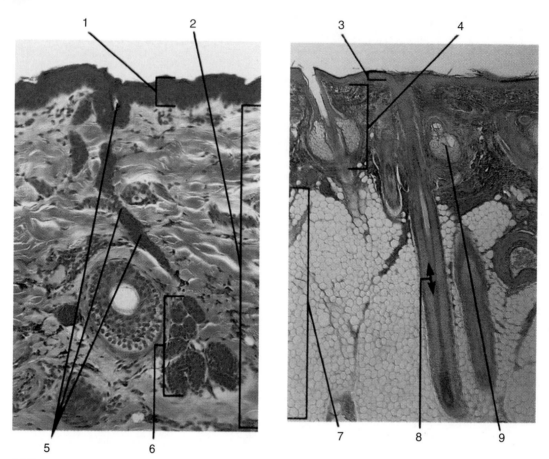

Figure 14.2

Relevant Terms	
_____ Dermis	_____ Hair follicle
_____ Dermis	_____ Hypodermis
_____ Duct of sweat gland	_____ Sebaceous gland
_____ Epidermis	_____ Sweat gland
_____ Epidermis	

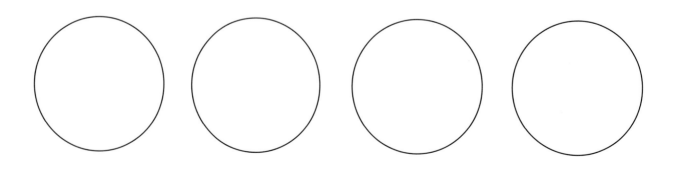

Section B. Assessments

1. T/F   The visible part of a hair is called the *follicle*.
2. T/F   Sebaceous glands produce the skin's oil, which is called *sebum*.
3. The part of the skin responsible for producing a set of fingerprints is the:
   a. stratum corneum.
   b. dermal papillae.
   c. stratum germinativum.
   d. subcutaneous layer.
4. The _____ is the small muscle responsible for hair movement.
   a. hair papilla
   b. sebaceous gland
   c. arrector pili
   d. hair root

Section C. Critical Thinking Problem

1. Considering the military analogy of the skin, what (if any) would be the related military components that are analogous to hair? pores? skin receptors? sebaceous glands? sweat glands?

Unit 5

Respiration, Nutrition, and Excretion

"The city is not a concrete jungle, it is a human zoo."

Desmond Morris

How does a city meet the needs of its citizens?

The human body consists of anywhere between 20-50 trillion cells, each of which requires certain conditions and components to live. The body maintains many of the conditions that cells need, such as temperature, by balancing a host of factors to keep the environment stable, a condition called *homeostasis*. Vital components, such as nutrients, water, and oxygen, must be introduced into the body continually. Furthermore, cellular processing of these nutrients produces waste and without its removal, rising amounts of waste will compromise the health of all cells.

Much like the cells in the body, citizens of a city have certain needs, such as food, water, shelter, electricity, sanitation, and transportation. Cities without these basic needs are rife with disease, malnutrition, and death. Even the most affluent nations can have broken cities where the government has failed to balance the needs of its citizens by ensuring a flow of goods into the city, the availability of power, and the removal of waste.

In this unit, we will explore the digestive, respiratory, and urinary systems and explore how each of these systems interacts with tissues to meet the vital needs of the cells, the citizens of the body.

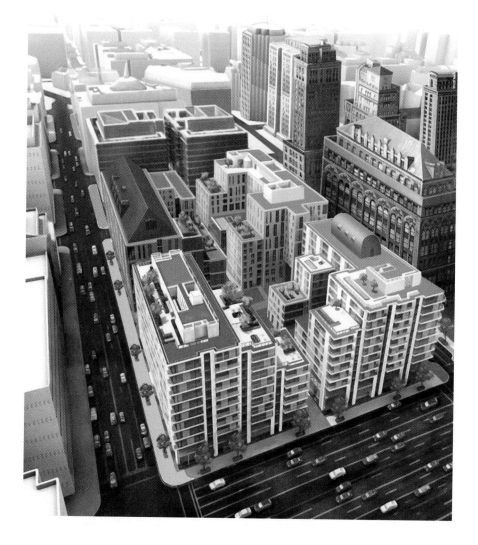

Exercise 15

The Digestive System

Overview

In the fifth century BC, many of the towns built in Greece were modeled after plans developed by Hippodamus, and included residential areas organized into blocks, large areas for public access, and wide main streets for easy transportation. Fresh water systems were created and drainage systems for sanitation were also installed. This design accommodated the center of Greek life, the agora, which was the heart of the city where goods were traded in markets.

Today's cities reflect the urbanization — the process in which higher percentages of citizens live in highly populated areas — of modern times. While some cities around the world have retained their distinct city centers for food markets, the agora has been widely replaced by grocery and department stores distributed throughout a city. Items are shipped into the network of stores through an extensive transport industry that includes truck, air, rail, and water transport.

In a similar vein, cells depend upon systems to deliver essential components directly to them. The digestion of food produces substances that can be absorbed into the bloodstream, and these 'goods' are delivered to regional tissues for further distribution to cells. In this exercise, you will explore the digestive system first by following the path of food through the body then by experiments with an enzyme that aids in the process of digestion.

Activity #1 — Digestive Organs

Introduction

The "tube-within-a-tube" body of animals, including humans, connects the mouth to the anus by a long gastrointestinal tract. Through the contraction of this muscular tube, food migrates through the body.

Consumed food is a like a truck carrying molecular goods into a city. Traveling along its route through the gastrointestinal tract, it makes various stops to deliver specific shipments as substances are absorbed from digested materials. And once emptied of all valuable content, it heads out of the city.

In this activity, you will investigate the organs of the digestive tract and study slide samples of important tissues.

Materials

Textbook
Models of the digestive system
Microscope
Slides of the stomach wall and small intestine.

Procedure

1. Review content in your textbook related to the digestive organs.

2. The gastrointestinal (GI) tract, or alimentary canal, is a muscular tube approximately 30 feet long that progresses from mouth to anus. Encased by the body, its interior is considered part of the external environment of the body. The process of digestion in the alimentary canal is similar to an assembly line — with substances moving along a one-way path and undergoing changes at each stage — but one that is geared to break down rather than construct materials. To gain a better understanding of the digestive organs that make up the canal and the accessory organs that support it, identify the vital organs and important features of the alimentary canal in Figure 15.2 in the Lab Report.

3. The wall of the alimentary canal participates in the movement of substances as well as secretion, digestion, and absorption. It consists of four concentric layers of muscular and connective tissue with blood vessels and nerve fibers in all but the innermost mucosa layer. Label the layers and important structures that make up the wall of the GI tract in Figure 15.3 in the Lab Report.

4. Use a microscope to view a prepared slide of the wall of the stomach and small intestine. Draw what you observe in the space provided in your lab report. Note the extra muscular layer in the stomach and comment on what its function is. Examine the structure of the villi in the small intestine and draw what you observe.

5. The digestive tract begins with the oral cavity, or the mouth, which contains the muscular tongue, a set of 32 teeth, and saliva-releasing salivary glands that begin the physical and chemical digestion of food through mastication. Locate the features of the oral cavity and support structures in Figure 15.4 in the Lab Report.

6. Posterior to the oral cavity is the fibromuscular pharynx or throat. Like the mouth, the pharynx is a part of the respiratory and digestive systems and directs solid, liquid, and gaseous substances to the correct path. While air takes the respiratory route, other substances are directed to the esophagus, a long muscular tube that guides substances, along with the aid of gravity, toward the stomach. Use Figure 15.5 in the Lab Report to find the important features of the pharynx and esophagus.

7. Inferior to the diaphragm, the stomach is a saclike organ that temporarily stores food while promoting physical digestion with muscular contraction and chemical digestion as food churns in a bath of hydrochloric acid. Review Figure 15.3 to familiarize yourself with the key features of the stomach.

8. The lower digestive tract begins with the small intestine at the duodenum, one of the most important sites in digestion as it receives substances from the pyloric end of the stomach. The duodenum extends into the jejunum, which transitions into the ileum to connect to the large intestine. All six meters of the coiled small intestine are suspended in the abdominal cavity by mesentery, allowing great motility to pass substances via muscular contraction. Along the lumen walls, fingerlike projections called *villi* increase the surface area for absorption of digested substances. Identify the key features of the small intestine in Figure 15.6 in the Lab Report.

9. The five-foot long large intestine emerges from the small intestine and is divided into (1) the ascending colon, where the appendix is attached, (2) the transverse colon, and (3) the descending colon that passes waste material into the rectum and on into the anus. Fecal matter is compacted through the small intestine as water is removed. Use Figure 15.7 in the Lab Report to place the correct anatomical terms of the large intestine in the spaces provided.

10. While food completes a one-way passage through the GI tract, a few important accessory organs outside of the alimentary canal play key roles in digestion, specifically at the site of the duodenum. Here, ducts that extend from the liver, gallbladder, and pancreas connect to release digestive enzymes and other materials. One of the most important functions of the liver is the production of bile, which may be temporarily stored in the gallbladder before draining into the common bile duct that converges with the pancreatic duct carrying other digestive enzymes. Label the features of the liver, gallbladder and pancreas in Figure 15.8 in the Lab Report.

Lab Report for 15.1

Section A. Activities for Digestive Organs

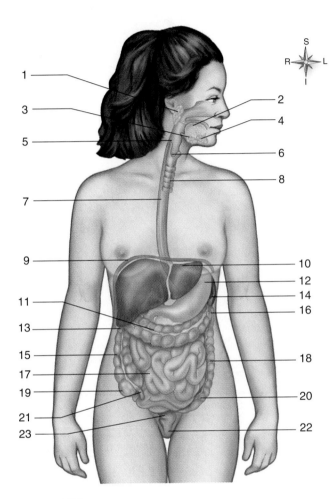

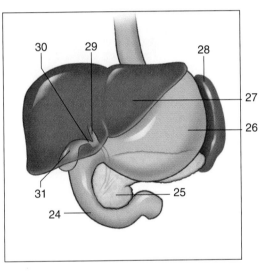

Figure 15.2

Relevant Terms		
_____ Anal canal	_____ Ilium	_____ Spleen
_____ Ascending colon	_____ Larynx	_____ Splenic flexure of color
_____ Cecum	_____ Liver	_____ Stomach
_____ Common hepatic duct	_____ Liver	_____ Stomach
_____ Cystic duct	_____ Pancreas	_____ Sublingual salivary gland
_____ Descending colon	_____ Parotid gland	_____ Submandibular salivary gland
_____ Diaphragm	_____ Pharynx	_____ Tongue
_____ Duodenum	_____ Rectum	_____ Trachea
_____ Gallbladder	_____ Sigmoid colon	_____ Transverse colon
_____ Hepatic flexure of colon	_____ Spleen	_____ Vermiform appendix

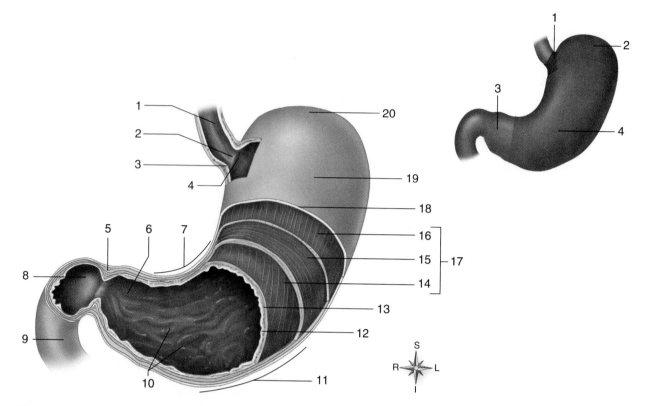

Figure 15.3

Relevant Terms		
Divisions of the Stomach	**Stomach**	
_____ Body	_____ Body of Stomach	_____ Longitudinal muscle layer
_____ Carida	_____ Cardia	_____ Lower esophageal sphincter
_____ Fundus	_____ Circular muscle layer	_____ Mucosa
_____ Pylorus	_____ Duodenal bulb	_____ Muscularis
	_____ Duodenum	_____ Oblique muscle layer
	_____ Esophagus	_____ Pyloric sphincter
	_____ Fundus	_____ Pylorus
	_____ Gastroesophageal opening	_____ Rugae
	_____ Greater curvature	_____ Serosa
	_____ Lesser curvature	_____ Submucosa

Use the following space to draw what you observe from the slide:

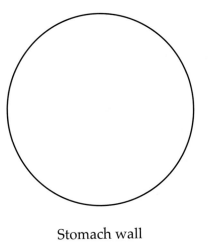

Stomach wall

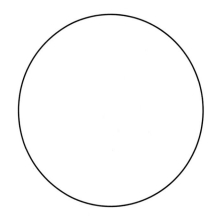

Intestinal wall

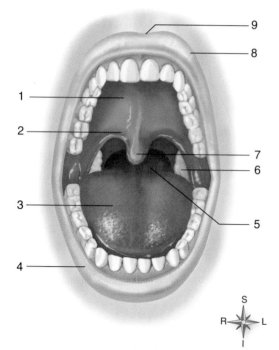

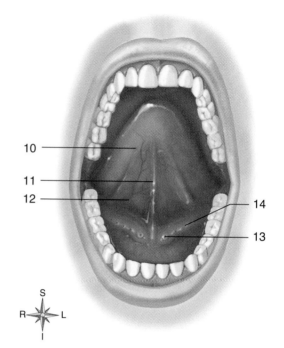

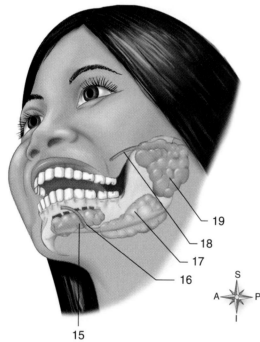

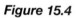

Figure 15.4

Relevant Terms
Oral Cavity
_____ Fauces
_____ Fimbriated fold
_____ Hard palate
_____ Lingual frenulum
_____ Lingual vein
_____ Lower lip
_____ Palatine tonsil
_____ Parotid duct
_____ Parotid gland
_____ Philtrum
_____ Soft palate
_____ Sublingual gland
_____ Sublingual gland
_____ Submandibular duct
_____ Submandibular duct
_____ Submandibular gland
_____ Tongue
_____ Upper lip
_____ Uvula

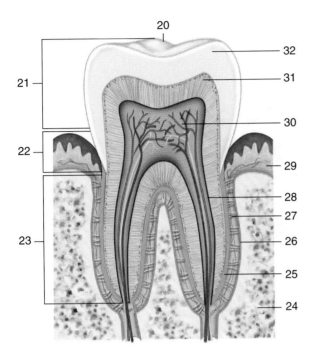

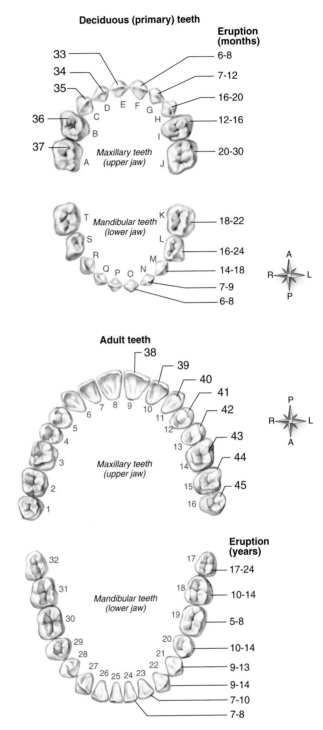

Deciduous (primary) teeth

Adult teeth

Figure 15.4 (con't)

Relevant Terms
Teeth
_____ Bone
_____ Canine
_____ Canine
_____ Cementum
_____ Central incisor
_____ Central incisor
_____ Crown
_____ Cusp
_____ Dentin
_____ Enamel
_____ First molar
_____ First molar
_____ First premolar
_____ Gingiva
_____ Lateral incisor
_____ Lateral incisor
_____ Neck
_____ Periodontal ligament
_____ Periodontal membrane
_____ Pulp cavity
_____ Root
_____ Root Canal
_____ Second molar
_____ Second molar
_____ Second premolar
_____ Third molar

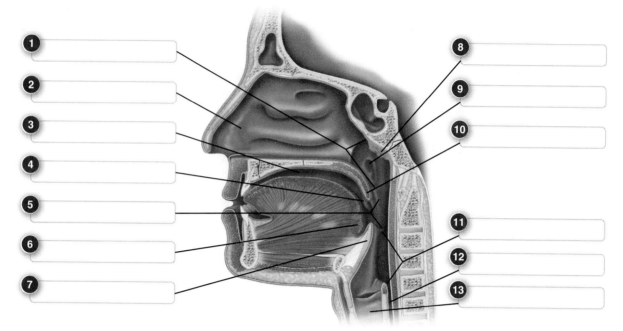

Figure 15.5

Relevant Terms	
Epiglottis	Oral cavity
Esophagus	Oropharynx
Eustachian tube	Palantine tonsil
Hypopharynx	Pharyngeal tonsil
Lingual tonsil	Trachea
Nasal cavity	Uvula
Nasopharynx	Venule

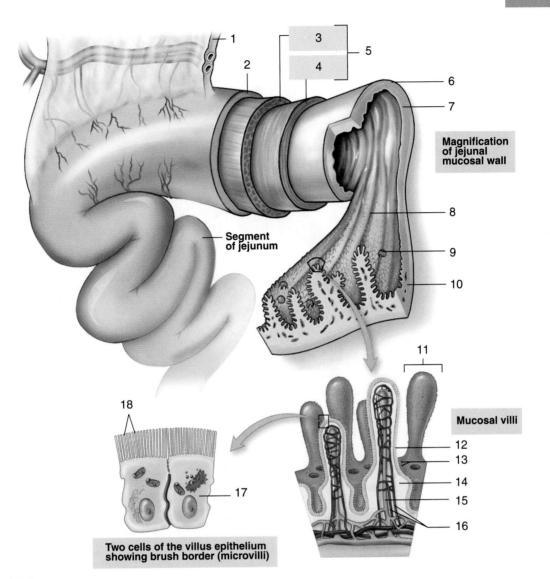

Magnification
of jejunal
mucosal wall

Segment
of jejunum

Mucosal villi

18

Two cells of the villus epithelium
showing brush border (microvilli)

Figure 15.6

Relevant Terms	
_____ Artery and vein	_____ Microvilli
_____ Circular muscle	_____ Microvilli
_____ Epithelial cell	_____ Mucosa
_____ Epithelium	_____ Mucosa
_____ Epithelium	_____ Muscularis
_____ Lacteal (lymph capillary)	_____ Plica (fold)
_____ Longitudinal muscle	_____ Serosa
_____ Lymph nodule	_____ Single villus
_____ Mesentery	_____ Submucosa

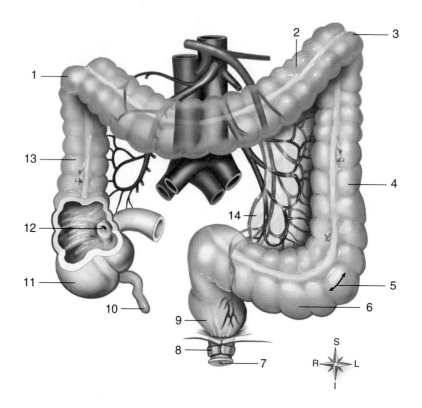

Figure 15.7

Relevant Terms	
_____ Anus	_____ Ileocecal valve
_____ Appendix	_____ Left colic (splenic) flexure
_____ Ascending colon	_____ Mesentery
_____ Cecum	_____ Rectum
_____ Descending colon	_____ Right colic (hepatic) flexure
_____ External anal sphincter	_____ Sigmoid colon
_____ Haustra	_____ Transverse colon

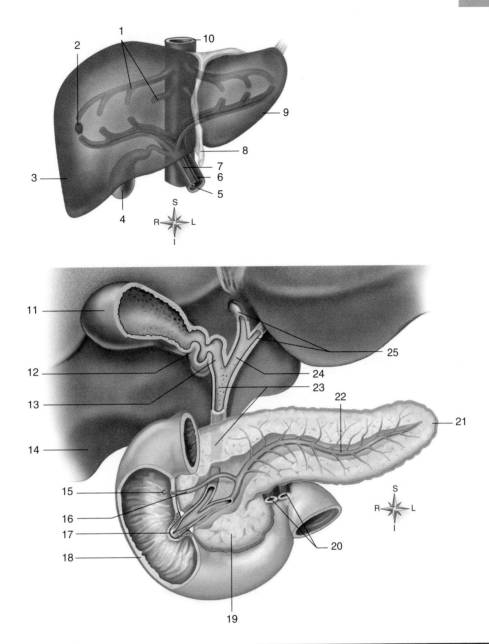

Figure 15.8

Relevant Terms		
Liver	**Gallbladder**	**Pancreas**
____ Bile duct	____ Common bile duct	____ Accessory pancreatic duct
____ Falciform ligament	____ Common hepatic duct	____ Duodenum
____ Gallbladder	____ Corpus	____ Head of pancreas
____ Hepatic artery	____ Cystic duct	____ Major duodenal papilla
____ Hepatic portal vein	____ Liver	____ Minor duodenal papilla
____ Hepatic veins	____ Neck of gallbladder	____ Pancreatic duct
____ Inferior vena cava	____ Right and left hepatic ducts	____ Superior mesenteric artery and vein
____ Left lobe		____ Tail of pancreas
____ Lobule		
____ Right lobe		

Section B. Assessments

1. T/F The pharynx is part of both the digestive and respiratory systems.
2. T/F The esophagus connects to the pyloric end of the stomach.
3. Which of the following is an accessory organ of the digestive system?
   a. gallbladder
   b. mouth
   c. villi
   d. ascending colon
4. What is the correct order of sections within the small intestine?
   a. duodenum, ileum, jejunum
   b. duodenum, jejunum, ileum
   c. jejunum, duodenum, ileum
   d. jejunum, ileum, duodenum
5. The wall of the alimentary canal participates in which of the following?
   a. secretion
   b. digestion
   c. absorption
   d. all of the above

2. The small intestine isn't smaller than the large intestine in terms of length but it does have a smaller diameter. The large intestine has three straight sections while the small intestine has many folds. How does the structure of each intestine relate to its function?

3. Considering the analogy of food being a truck delivering goods, at what point is the truck "empty"?

Section C. Critical Thinking Problems

1. While the lower digestive tract involves many folds and turns, the upper digestive tract is fairly straight, especially the pharynx and esophagus. Why would it be detrimental for these structures to be folded or curved?

Activity #2 — Digestive Enzymes

Introduction

Retail stores employ a variety of people to unload pallets from trucks, track inventory, and stock shelves for consumers. While these jobs are often unheralded, they are essential for citizens of a city to conveniently purchase goods. It could be said that these employees are as valuable to consumerism as enzymes are to digestion, in that enzymes unpack molecular inventory from food. Enzymes are large molecules that are able to make or break chemical bonds and in this light, they are the unheralded workers of digestion.

To delve into the action of enzymes in digestion at a deeper level, we will investigate one of the digestive enzymes responsible for the breakdown of polysaccharides in food, amylase.

Materials

Textbook
Stethoscopes
Alcohol swabs
Paper cups
Stopwatch or timer
Saltine crackers (preferably unsalted)
Test tubes
Test tube rack
1% soluble starch solution
1% maltose solution
Pancreatin powder
Spatulas
Distilled water
Lugol's reagent
Benedict's reagent
Disposable 1-mL droppers or pipettes
Hot plates
Ice-water bath
Warm-water bath (at 37° C)
Beakers
Thermometers

Before You Begin

- *Your instructor will demonstrate correct laboratory procedures for the proper handling and disposal of chemicals.*
- *Be sure that you are not chewing gum or candy before or during the lab as it can affect your sense of taste for this first activity.*

Procedure

1. Review content in your textbook related to digestion and digestive enzymes.

The Effect of Amylase in Saliva

2. Both physical and chemical digestion begins in the mouth through the process of mastication and hydrolysis of starches, respectively. The hydrolyzing enzyme, α-amylase, is secreted by the salivary glands as part of saliva, and it breaks down starches into maltose when it is around body temperature. Because enzymes are sensitive to heat, amylase will not break down starch at cold temperatures and at hot temperatures, amylase will denature.

3. To detect α-amylase in saliva, take a bite of a saltine cracker and start the timer. Continue to chew the cracker until the flavor of the cracker changes by becoming sweeter. The sweetness is from maltose, which has been hydrolyzed from the long polysaccharides of starch. Maltose is a disaccharide that is about half as sweet as glucose.

4. Record the time interval in your lab report.

Opening of the Cardioesophageal Sphincter

1. Swallowing passes substances down through the esophagus to the cardioesophageal sphincter, which controls how much and when food enters the stomach. You will listen to the opening of this sphincter by listening to a subject drink a mouthful of water.

2. Fill a cup with water for the subject to drink.

3. Obtain a stethoscope and clean the earpieces with alcohol swabs.

4. Place the earpieces in your ears and place the diaphragm or bell of the stethoscope on a subject's stomach about an inch lower than the xiphoid process and approximately half an inch to the left.

5. The subject should swallow a mouthful of water, at which point you will hear two sounds and you will determine the approximate time interval between them. The first is the water hitting the cardioesophageal sphincter. The second sound will be the opening of the sphincter, allowing water to enter the stomach (it will have a gurgling sound). The sphincter opens in response to the involuntary muscular contraction of the esophagus that aids in driving consumed substances toward the stomach, which is known as the *peristaltic wave*.

6. Record the time interval in your lab report.

The Action of Amylase on Starch

7. The pancreas also secretes amylase, which helps to break down remaining polysaccharides passing from the stomach into maltose. Maltose is then broken down by other enzymes into glucose, which can then be absorbed through the small intestine and into the blood.

8. To test whether amylase is present in an extract of pancreatic secretions, and to determine the temperature range for amylase function, you will investigate whether pancreatin powder can break down starch at three different temperatures. This is done best by detecting both the disappearance of starch in the presence of the extract as well as the production of maltose. Starch can be detected using a chemical called *Lugol's reagent* and maltose can be tested by using *Benedict's reagent*. Since both reagents have special conditions for their use and a positive result is confirmed visually, you will first perform a test run with each reagent to observe what a positive and negative result look like for each.

9. *Lugol's test:* To a test tube, add 2 mL of distilled water and a few drops of Lugol's reagent. Lugol's reagent is a solution containing iodine, which has a dark orange-brown color, so a few drops dissolved into water should produce a light orange solution.

10. To a second test tube, add 2 mL of 1% starch solution and a few drops of Lugol's reagent. In the presence of starch, the iodine in the Lugol's reagent forms a complex with starch that produces a dark blue-to-black colored solution.

11. Label the test tubes "L–" and "L+" or other appropriate labeling to indicate the negative and positive Lugol results, respectively. Place the two test tubes aside for later reference. Record your observations in your lab report.

12. *Benedict's test:* To a test tube, add 2 mL of distilled water and 2 mL of Benedict's reagent.

13. To a second test tube, add 2 mL of 1% maltose solution and 2 mL of Benedict's reagent.

14. Place each tube in a beaker of boiling water. After 3 minutes, remove each tube and place them on the test tube rack to cool. Benedict's reagent is blue, so a light blue color should be obtained in the first test tube as a negative result. The presence of sugar is detected when the solution changes color, usually to green yellow, orange or red, depending upon the concentration of sugar.

15. Label the test tubes "B–" and "B+" or other appropriate labeling to indicate the negative and positive Benedict results, respectively. Place the two test tubes aside for later reference. Record your observations in your lab report.

16. *Testing the pancreatin powder:* You will now use Lugol's and Benedict's reagents to test the enzymatic activity of pancreatin powder. To each of 8 test tubes, add 2 mL of 1% starch solution. Using a spatula, add a pea-sized amount of the powder to each of the test tubes. Assign labels to each of the tubes with your initials and a number and letter afterward (1L and 1B, 2L and 2B, etc.) that will correspond to the following:
    a. Place two test tubes in an ice-water bath (about 0° C)
    b. Place two test tubes on the rack at room temperature (varies, but usually about 20-25° C)

c. Place two test tubes in the warm-water bath (37° C)

d. Place two test tubes in a boiling-water bath. (100° C)

17. Allow the test tubes to remain at these temperatures for 10-15 minutes. Be sure to remove the test tubes in the hot-water bath before the solutions boil down below 0.5 mL.

18. Test each of the solutions labeled with an "L" by adding a few drops of Lugol's reagent to each. Record and analyze your results in your lab report.

19. Test each of the solutions labeled with a "B" by adding a few drops of Benedict's reagent to each. Place each tube in a beaker of boiling water. After 3 minutes, remove each tube and place them on the rack to cool. Record and analyze your results in your lab report.

Section A. Activities for Digestive Enzymes

Time interval between the beginning of mastication and a sweet taste:	_____ s
Time interval between water reaching the cardioesophageal sphincter and its opening:	_____ s
Observations when testing Lugol's reagent:	
Observations when testing Benedict's reagent:	
Observations of the test solutions in the ice-water bath:	
Observations of the test solutions at room temperature:	
Observations of the test solutions in the warm-water bath:	
Observations of the test solutions in the boiling-water bath:	
Analysis of the enzymatic activity of pancreatin powder:	

Section B. Assessments

1. T/F The end product of amylase digestion is monosaccharides.
2. T/F When the cardioesophageal sphincter opens, food passes into the duodenum.
3. Where is amylase produced?
   a. stomach
   b. salivary glands
   c. pancreas
   d. both b and c above

Section C. Critical Thinking Problems

1. Name two other foods which might taste sweet after chewing them for a while. Relate any experiences you've had that can confirm the action of amylase when consuming these foods.

2. In light of this lab activity, what would happen to enzymes in your cells if you experienced hypothermia? What about hyperthermia?

Exercise 16

The Respiratory System

Overview

Consider the role that oxygen plays in the body. Oxygen absorbed in the lungs enters the bloodstream and is distributed throughout the body. The only structures in the body that require oxygen are the mitochondria in cells, and they need oxygen only for the last step of cellular respiration. Yet, this one step controls the primary means of energy production in the body, justifying the body's need for such a large system to support respiration. Without oxygen, metabolic processes shut down rapidly.

Considering the analogy of a city being like the human body, which component of a city is similar to oxygen, in that its absence brings everything to a standstill? Electricity.

In this unit, we will explore the organs that make up the respiratory system and then study the process of respiration in more depth.

Activity #1 — Respiratory Organs

Introduction

Similar to the digestive system, the respiratory system includes a set of organs involved in the transport and absorption of materials into the body. But there are significant differences between these systems:

1. The material flowing through the respiratory system is air, which is a gas, unlike the liquid or solid materials passing through in the digestive system. Therefore, a different mechanism is required to "ingest" and "excrete" materials, which is respiration.

2. Only one substance, oxygen, is absorbed in the process of respiration and only one waste substance, carbon dioxide, is produced.

3. The passage of air in the respiratory system is bidirectional, which allows for the system to absorb the necessary amount of oxygen when air flows in (during inhalation) and release carbon dioxide to flow out with the excess oxygen left in the air (during exhalation).

> **Materials**
>
> Textbook
> Models of the respiratory system
> Slides of the trachea, normal lung tissue, and
> damaged lung tissue (from smoking)

Procedure

1. Review content in your textbook related to the respiratory organs.
2. Use a microscope to view prepared slides of the wall of the trachea and lung. In the trachea, identify the various tissues layers. For the slide of lung tissue, identify the bronchiole and alveoli. Compare the slides of the healthy lung tissue to the damaged lung tissue. Draw what you observe in the space provided in your Lab Report.
3. The respiratory system is an enclosed system that partially overlaps with the digestive system. The upper respiratory tract shares the oral cavity and pharynx with the digestive tract, while the nasal cavity is also a source of air intake. The lower respiratory tract diverges from the GI tract at the larynx as air flows into the trachea and enters the lungs, where oxygen is absorbed and carbon dioxide is released. To gain an understanding of the respiratory organs, identify the vital organs and important features in Figure 16.1 in the Lab Report.
4. The upper respiratory tract begins at the nasal cavity, which consists of a series of bony plates, covered with a ciliated epithelium, which forms passageways for the inflow of air through the nostrils, or anterior nares. The oral cavity, which can also be an intake for air, converges with the nasal cavity and extends at the pharynx before the divergence at the larynx, commonly referred to as the *voice box*. Label the key features of the upper respiratory tract in Figure 16.2 in the Lab Report.
5. The lower respiratory tract includes the trachea, or windpipe, which is an approximately 4.5-inch long tube of smooth muscle containing cartilaginous rings for support. The trachea diverges into two primary bronchi encased by the lungs. These bronchi further divide into secondary and tertiary bronchi with further branching forming bronchioles that terminate with alveolar ducts. Like grapes on a vine, the 300 million alveoli in the lungs are the site of gas exchange. Identify the key features of the lower respiratory tract in Figure 16.3 in the Lab Report.

Lab Report for 16.1

Section A. Activities for Respiratory Organs

Use the following space to draw what you observe from the slide:

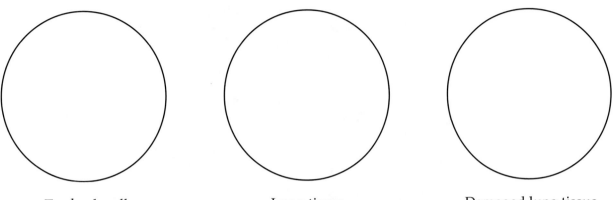

Tracheal wall   Lung tissue   Damaged lung tissue

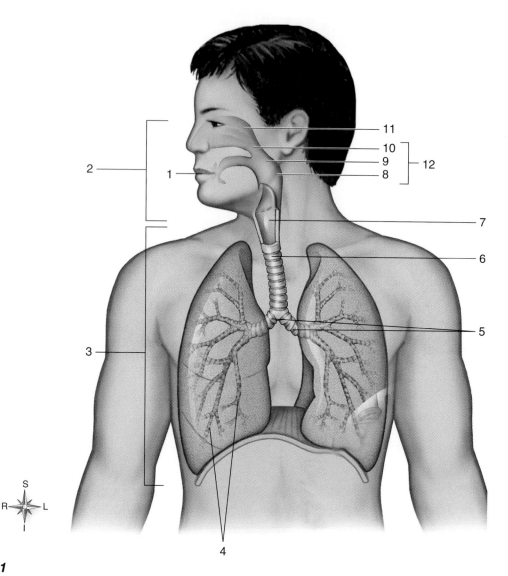

Figure 16.1

Relevant Terms	
_____ Bronchioles	_____ Nasopharynx
_____ Laryngopharynx	_____ Oral cavity
_____ Larynx	_____ Oropharynx
_____ Left and right primary bronchi	_____ Pharynx
_____ Lower respiratory tract	_____ Trachea
_____ Nasal cavity	_____ Upper respiratory tract

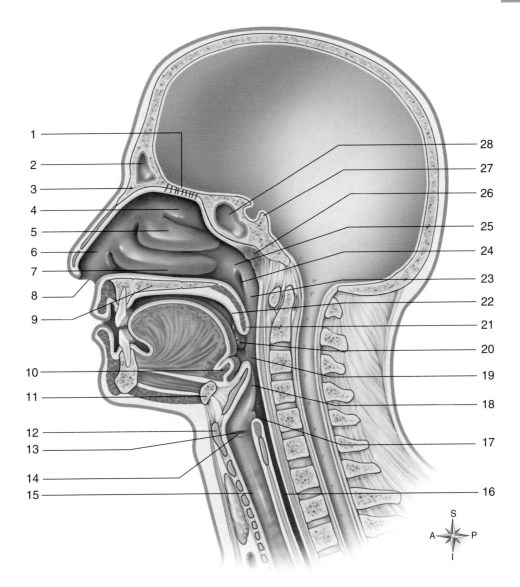

Figure 16.2

Relevant Terms		
_____ Anterior naris	_____ Larynx	_____ Sella turcica
_____ Cranial cavity	_____ Lingual tonsil	_____ Soft palate
_____ Cribriform plate of ethmoid bone	_____ Middle nasal concha of ethmoid	_____ Sphenoid sinus
_____ Epiglottis	_____ Nasal bone	_____ Superior nasal concha of ethmoid
_____ Esophagus	_____ Nasopharynx	_____ Thyroid cartilage
_____ Frontal sinus	_____ Opening of auditory (eustachian) tube	_____ Trachea
_____ Hard palate	_____ Oropharynx	_____ Uvula
_____ Hyoid bone	_____ Palatine tonsil	_____ Vestibule
_____ Inferior concha	_____ Pharyngeal tonsil (adenoids)	_____ Vocal cords
_____ Laryngopharynx	_____ Posterior naris	

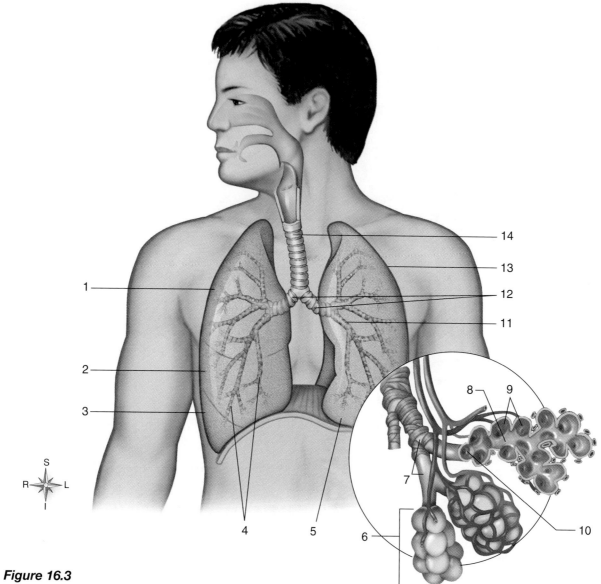

Figure 16.3

Relevant Terms			
_____ Alveolar duct		_____ Right inferior lobe	
_____ Alveolar sac		_____ Right middle lobe	
_____ Alveoli		_____ Right superior lobe	
_____ Left inferior lobe		_____ Secondary bronchi	
_____ Left superior lobe		_____ Terminal bronchiole	
_____ Primary bronchi		_____ Tertiary bronchi	
_____ Respiratory bronchiole		_____ Trachea	

Section B. Assessments

1. T/F   The trachea is the beginning of the upper respiratory tract.
2. The larynx is also known as the:
    a. Adam's apple.
    b. voice box.
    c. windpipe.
    d. COPD.
3. The site of gas exchange in the lung is at the:
    a. primary bronchi.
    b. secondary bronchi.
    c. bronchioles.
    d. alveolar ducts.

Section C. Critical Thinking Problem

1. The trachea is supported by smooth muscle and cartilaginous rings. These cartilaginous rings are C-shaped. Can you explain the purpose of these cartilaginous rings and why they do not surround the entire trachea?

Activity #2 — Breathing

Introduction

If you hold your breath, oxygen molecules will flow into your lungs by diffusing through the air and be absorbed by the alveoli. However, the amount absorbed is not nearly enough to meet the demands of all the cells in the body. Ultimately, the process of breathing is about increasing the rate of airflow in and out of the lungs, so that the rate of absorption of oxygen at the alveoli is adequate for the body's needs. When the demand for oxygen is increased during strenuous activity, breath rate increases and the lungs expand to larger volumes to ensure that oxygen demands are met. Extreme physical activity can result in an insufficient oxygen intake to keep up with the demand from muscle cells. This results in cells kicking into anaerobic metabolism that causes a rapid buildup of lactic acid.

The electrical supply to a city is similar to the oxygen present in the lungs. When energy demands increase, power plants must increase the flow of electricity. During peak summer temperatures when electricity use is high, brownouts and blackouts can occur due to the demand being greater than the supply.

In this activity, you will investigate aspects of pulmonary ventilation, commonly known as *breathing*, as well as specific pulmonary volumes and capacities.

Materials

Textbook
Spirometer
Clean mouthpieces

Before You Begin

- *Your instructor will demonstrate the proper use of the spirometer for each of the measurements you will take in this activity.*

Procedure

1. Review content in your textbook related to external respiration.

   The process of respiration is complicated: a mixture of gases is transported in and out of the system and the flow is bi-directional. The overall amount of gas exchange depends on the surface area of the alveoli and the volume of air that is present in the lungs. To properly describe pulmonary capacity, you will use the spirometer to measure different pulmonary volumes in the following activities. The spirometer measures air flow in and out of the device, but it cannot measure the total volume of your lungs. You will have to determine the volumes and capacities of respiration in stages based on your total lung capacity indicated in Appendix A. To help you understand the relationship between these volumes and capacities, study Figure 16.4.

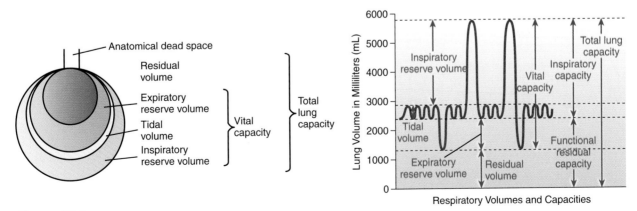

Figure 16.4

Pulmonary Volumes and Capacities

2. *Tidal volume (TV):* the volume of air (approximately 500 mL) moving in and out of the respiratory system in one normal breath or respiratory cycle. Measure your TV using the spirometer and record your results in your lab report.

3. *Expiratory reserve volume (ERV):* the volume of air (about 1,100 mL) that can be expelled after a normal exhalation. Note: the lungs are not completely emptied of air after the ERV is exhaled. The 1,200 mL of air remaining in the lungs is called the *residual volume (RV)* and cannot be measured with a spirometer. Measure your ERV using the spirometer and record your results in your lab report.

4. *Vital capacity (VC):* the volume of air that can be expelled after taking the deepest breath possible. Measure your VC using the spirometer and record your results in your lab report.

5. Using these values, it is possible to calculate other volumes and capacities:
   a. *Inspiratory reserve volume (IRV):* the volume of air (about 3,000 mL) that is inhaled above the tidal volume. Calculate this value by subtracting the tidal volume (TV) and the expiratory reserve volume (ERV) from the vital capacity (VC) and record the result in your lab report.
   b. *Inspiratory capacity (IC):* the volume of air (about 3,500 mL) that is inhaled in a deep breath after exhalation. Calculate this value by adding the tidal volume (TV) to the inspiratory reserve volume (IRV) and record the result in your lab report.
   c. *Functional residual capacity (FRC):* the volume of air (about 2,300 mL) remaining in the lungs after a normal breath (that is, the tidal volume). Calculate this value by adding the residual volume, which is 1,200 mL, to the expiratory reserve volume (ERV) and record the result in your lab report.

The Effect of Exercise

6. Repeat steps 3-6 after exercising for 2-5 minutes (running in place, jumping rope, etc.).

Lab Report for 16.2

Section A. Activities for Breathing

	Formula	At rest (mL)	After exercising (mL)
Measure:			
Tidal volume (TV)			
Expiratory reserve volume (ERV)			
Vital capacity (VC)			
Calculate:			
Inspiratory reserve volume (IRV)	IRV = VC − TV − ERV		
Inspiratory capacity (IC)	IC = TV + IRV		
Functional residual capacity (FRC)	FRC = ERV + 1,200 mL		

1. What is the effect of exercise on each of the pulmonary volumes and capacities?

Section B. Assessments

1. T/F   During inhalation, the volume of the chest cavity is reduced.
2. T/F   Vital capacity contains the residual volume.
3. Breathing is also known as:
    a. total capacity.
    b. internal respiration.
    c. external respiration.
    d. pulmonary ventilation.
4. The volume of air moving into and out of the lung during regular breathing is:
    a. vital capacity.
    b. tidal volume.
    c. residual volume.
    d. inspiratory reserve volume.

Section C. Critical Thinking Problem

1. Would it be possible to develop related volumes and capacities for the digestive system? Explain.

Exercise 17

The Urinary System

Overview

Modern cities require extensive sanitation and waste disposal programs. In the US, the average person produces 100 gallons of urine and a half a ton of feces per year. All of that waste is enormously detrimental to the cells in the body if it is not removed, and so, the body has multiple ways of excreting waste. As seen in the previous exercises of this unit, fecal material is released through the digestive system and carbon dioxide is exhaled through the respiratory system. While the integumentary system can remove excess water and electrolytes, excretion is not its primary role. The burden falls upon the urinary system to remove the nitrogenous compounds, toxins, electrolytes, and excess water that would be detrimental to the body if allowed to accumulate.

In this exercise, you will investigate the organs of the urinary system and conduct an analysis of urine as a diagnostic of urinary system health.

Activity #1 — Urinary Organs

Introduction

Wastewater treatment plants use various forms of filtration to remove large and small components from sewage. After large components are removed, lower-density materials such as fats can be skimmed off the top and any sedimentation can be pumped away. Bacteria may be used to consume organic substances and then are filtered off and/or destroyed by disinfecting agents, such as ultraviolet light or chlorine.

In the urinary system, the kidneys serve as the main treatment plants of the blood. You will explore the kidneys in the following activity.

Materials

Textbook
Models of the urinary system
Slide of the renal cortex
Microscope

Procedure

1. Review content in your textbook related to the urinary organs.
2. Use a microscope to view a prepared slide of the renal cortex and compare it to Figure 17.1. Draw what you observe in the space provided in your lab report.

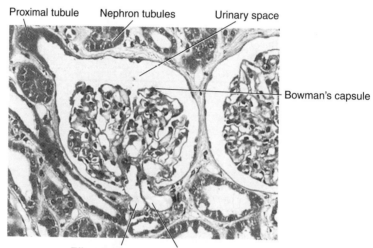

Proximal tubule   Nephron tubules   Urinary space

Bowman's capsule

Efferent artery   Afferent artery

Figure 17.1

3. The urinary system is responsible for more than just eliminating waste substances from the blood. It also maintains extracellular and intracellular fluid volume, and the proper pH of blood by balancing the electrolyte and water content of blood. It performs its duties by processing the blood in the kidneys, which remove nitrogenous wastes and delivers them to the bladder for temporary storage until they can be released through the urethra. To get a better understanding of the urinary system, label the appropriate structures in Figure 17.2 in the Lab Report.

4. The primary organs of the urinary tract are the two fist-sized kidneys, each containing about 1 million functional units called *nephrons* that filter blood. In a nephron, the renal corpuscle consists of glomerular capillaries embedded in Bowman's capsule. Waste compounds and electrolytes are fil- tered from the blood first in the glomerulus then in Bowman capsule. The resulting filtrate is passed to the renal tubule for processing where reabsorption of vital materials can occur and other waste materials can be added, then the remaining liquid drains into the collecting duct and passes to the ureter as urine. Label the important features of the kidney in Figure 17.3 and the nephron in Figure 17.4 in the Lab Report.

5. The urinary bladder is a muscular sac that is a temporary reservoir of urine, which can expand depending on the volume of urine present. In men, the bladder is located anterior to the rectum and superior to the prostate while in women, the bladder is located anterior to the vagina. Identify the key features of the bladder in men and women using Figure 17.5 in the Lab Report.

Section A. Activities for Urinary Organs

Use the following space to draw what you observe from the slide:

Renal cortex

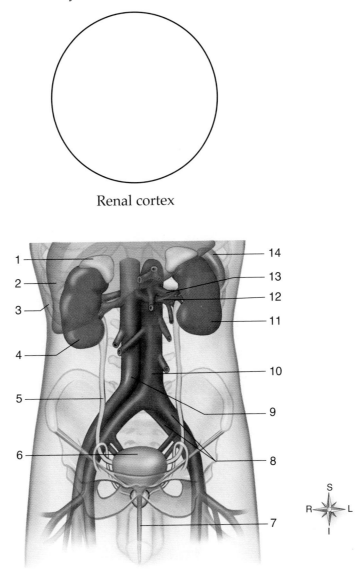

Figure 17.2

Relevant Terms	
_____ Abdominal aorta	_____ Renal vein
_____ Adrenal gland	_____ Right kidney
_____ Common iliac artery and vein	_____ Spleen
_____ Inferior vena cava	_____ Twelfth rib
_____ Left kidney	_____ Ureter
_____ Liver	_____ Urethra
_____ Renal artery	_____ Urinary bladder

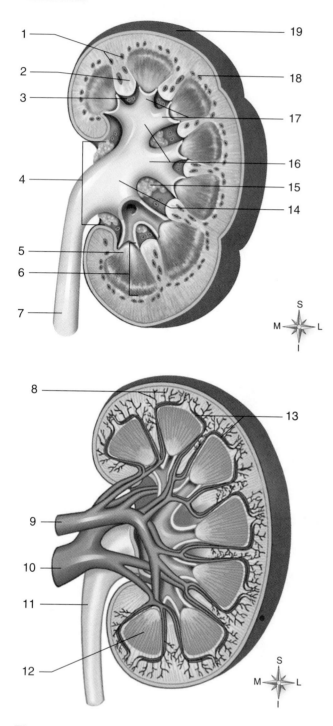

Figure 17.3

Relevant Terms
_____ Arcuate arteries and veins
_____ Capsule
_____ Cortex
_____ Fat
_____ Hilum
_____ Interlobular arteries
_____ Interlobular arteries and veins
_____ Major calyces
_____ Medulla
_____ Minor calyces
_____ Renal artery
_____ Renal column
_____ Renal papilla of pyramid
_____ Renal pelvis
_____ Renal pyramid
_____ Renal sinus
_____ Renal vein
_____ Ureter
_____ Ureter

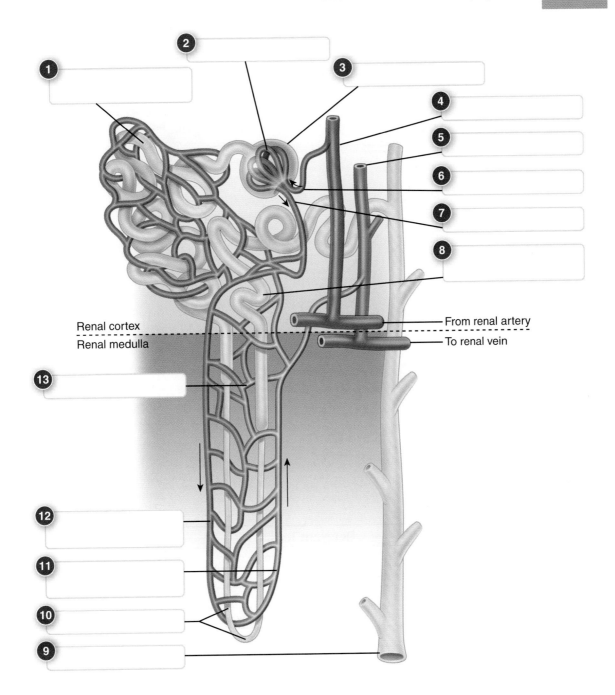

1

2

3

4

5

6

7

8

Renal cortex

Renal medulla

From renal artery

To renal vein

13

12

11

10

9

Figure 17.4

Relevant Terms	
Afferent arteriole	Glomerular capsule
Ascending limb of the nephron loop	Glomerulus
Collecting duct	Interlobular artery
Descending limb of the nephron loop	Interlobular vein
Distal convoluted tubule	Peritubular capillary
Efferent arteriole	Proximal convoluted tubule

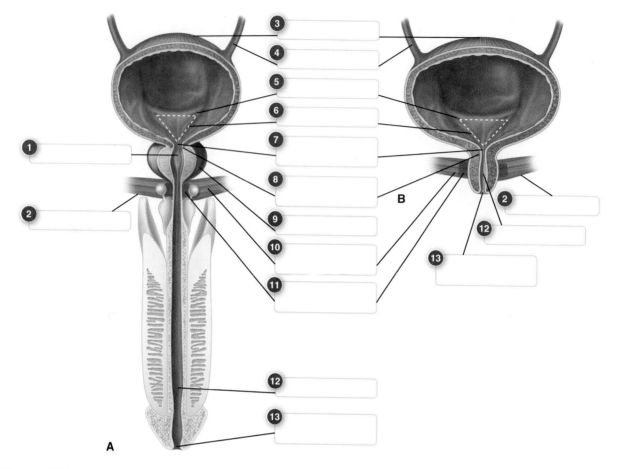

Figure 17.5

Relevant Terms	
External urethral orifice	Trigone
External urethral sphincter	Ureter
Internal urethral orifice	Urethra
Internal urethral sphincter	Urethral orifices
Pelvic floor	Urinary bladder
Prostate gland	Urogenital diaphragm
Prostatic urethra	

Section B. Assessments

1. T/F   The glomerulus catches filtrate from the Bowman capsule.
2. Which of the following do the kidneys do?
    a. Receive 10% of the blood pumped from the heart
    b. Help maintain proper blood pH
    c. Flow filtered blood back to the heart
    d. Break down lipids absorbed in the digestive tract
3. Urine is released from the body through the:
    a. ureter.
    b. urethra.
    c. nephron.
    d. urinary bladder.

Section C. Critical Thinking Problem

1. The kidneys filter only about 20% of the cardiac output per minute. If the kidneys were incorporated directly into the cardiovascular system so that 100% of blood could be filtered with each heartbeat, would this be superior to what is naturally found in the human body?

Activity #2 — Urinalysis

Introduction

The Great Pacific Garbage Patch, a collection of trash approximately twice the size of Texas floating in the Pacific Ocean, consists primarily of plastic dumped from ships and washed out to sea from beaches around the world. Scientists have discovered that the patch is leeching toxic chemicals into the ocean. Furthermore, the presence of mercury and other toxins in the ocean points to a failure to enforce regulations aimed at maintaining the health of the world's greatest resource.

Similarly, an analysis of a person's urine can reveal what is being consumed, as many drug users discover during drug testing, as well as the state of health. Hence, health practitioners have used urinalysis as a diagnostic tool for disease when other symptoms are present.

In this activity, you will analyze packaged urine samples to gain insight into what a urinalysis can reveal.

Materials

Textbook
Packaged normal and abnormal urine samples
Multitest strip (Multistix 10SG)
Test tubes
Centrifuge
Centrifuge tubes
Disposable pipette or dropper
Microscope
Microscope slides
Sedistain

Procedure

1. Review content in your textbook related to urine composition and urinalysis.
2. Urine composition varies with diet and physical activity, but can also provide insight into the functioning of the kidneys and other organs. You will analyze samples of urine, which may be normal or abnormal, depending on what is available. Each sample can be analyzed in three different ways: physical characterization, chemical analysis, and microscopic examination.

Physical Characterization

3. *Color:* As urine consists of approximately 95% water, one of the simplest observations that can be made is the color of the urine, which should be a pale yellow to amber color. A variety of color aberrations can occur that may serve as a warning for further testing, such as a red to dark brown, which may indicate blood present or a greenish color, which may indicate bile. At the same time, other factors such as diet and exercise can affect the color of the urine without signaling any disease. Therefore, urine color plays a secondary role as a diagnostic tool. Observe the color of the urine sample and record your results in your lab report.
4. *Transparency:* Normal urine is clear, though it may have a slight cloudiness, especially if it has been sitting. Cloudy urine may result from the presence of inorganic salts, fat globules, mucus, microbes, or epithelial cells. Observe the transparency of the urine sample and record your results in your lab report.

Chemical Analysis

5. While chemical components can be tested one at a time, modern test strips have been developed that provide a rapid diagnostic assessment of the chemical composition of urine. Typically, these strips are dipped into the urine sample for a length of time and then removed for analysis. Follow the instructions provided for your particular test strip and record the results for the following tests in your lab report:
   a. *Specific gravity:* Specific gravity is a measure of the density of a solution compared to water, which provides the solute concentration of the sample. Urine normally has a specific gravity ranging from 1.001 to 1.030. Higher values will indicate more concentrated urine due to dehydration while lower numbers generally indicate excessive fluid intake.

b. *pH*: Urine acidity or pH is typically between 4.6 to 8.0, depending upon the diet, though it is typically nearer to 6.0. A pH that is low can indicate starvation or dehydration while a high pH may occur in urinary infections.

c. *Glucose*: Glucose is typically not found in urine though it may appear after a high-carbohydrate meal or may be glycosuria, as a result of diabetes mellitus.

d. *Protein*: As macromolecules, proteins do not pass into the urine. However, the smaller albumin proteins may pass into the urine after strenuous exercise. Prolonged presence of protein in urine may indicate kidney disease.

e. *Ketone*: Ketone formation occurs during fat metabolism, but if the diet lacks sufficient carbohydrates, such as during starvation or a special diet, ketones may pass into the urine.

f. *Bilirubin*: When RBCs break down in the liver, bilirubin is released from hemoglobin. However, if a liver disorder is present, higher concentrations of bilirubins may occur.

g. *Urobilinogen*: The natural breakdown of bilirubins produced the yellow urochrome, which is responsible for urine's color, but an excess amount may indicate liver disease.

h. *Occult blood*: Small amounts of hemoglobin from RBCs can be present in the urine without changing its color. This hidden or occult hemoglobin may indicate kidney infection or the presence of kidney stones damaging the urinary tract.

i. *Leukocytes*: Though small amounts of WBCs in urine are normal, increased levels may signal a urinary tract infection.

j. *Nitrites*: The presence of nitrites can signal the presence of bacteria along the urinary tract.

Microscopic Examination (skip if urine is synthetic)

6. Urine sediment can be examined for the presence of cells, crystals, or other materials that have sloughed off from the urinary tract. To concentrate sediments, stir or shake the urine sample (to suspend any sedimentation) and transfer 10 mL of urine into a centrifuge tube.

7. Insert the centrifuge tube into the centrifuge. Ensure that it is properly balanced before turning it on. Have your instructor check it before you start.

8. Spin the sample for 5 minutes.

9. Squeeze the bulb of a disposable pipette or dropper and carefully lower the tip into the urine. When the tip is at the bottom, carefully draw up a small amount of sedimentation. Place one drop of the sample onto a microscope slide. Add a drop of Sedistain. Place a coverslip on the slide.

10. Examine the slide using the microscope and compare what you observe to the representative illustrations of sediment components in Figure 17.6. Sketch your observations in your lab report.

CELLS

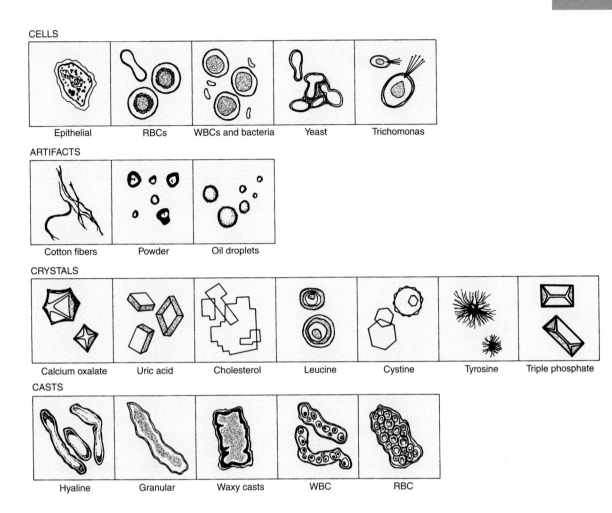

ARTIFACTS

CRYSTALS

CASTS

Figure 17.6

Lab Report for 17.2

Section A. Activities for Urinalysis

For the urine sample you analyzed, describe the results you obtained:

Characteristic	Results
Color:	
Transparency:	
Specific gravity:	
pH:	
Glucose:	
Protein:	
Ketone:	
Bilirubins:	
Urobilinogen:	
Occult blood:	
Leukocytes:	
Nitrites:	

Sketch your observations from the sediment:

Section B. Assessments

1. T/F   Discolored urine is always a sign of disease.
2. Glucose in the blood may be a sign of:
   a. diabetes mellitus.
   b. strenuous exercise.
   c. fat metabolism.
   d. bacteria in the urinary tract.
3. Urine that appears cloudy may contain excess:
   a. mucus.
   b. fat globules.
   c. inorganic salts.
   d. all of the above.

Section C. Critical Thinking Problem

1. Imagine a company develops a series of consumable, over-the-counter dyes that change urine to certain colors to indicate if disease is present. How might this be beneficial? What kind of response might average people have to this type of at-home test?

Unit 6

Reproduction and Development

We, that is our brains, are separate and independent enough from our genes to rebel against them. …we do so in a small way every time we use contraception.

Richard Dawkins, *The Selfish Gene*

Is our DNA the Constitution of our bodies?

Freedom can be defined as the ability to think and act unhindered by restraints imposed by anything other than the will. It is one of the most, if not *the* most, important factors in how we value living in the world today. When we look for examples of what being free looks like, nature often serves as the inspiration, simply because animals go about their lives in the absence of forces that deny freedom, such as political oppression, economic inequality, social injustice, religious intolerance, or censorship. This leads to a belief that if society demonstrated the kind of harmony seen in nature, we would have freedom for all.

Unfortunately, this view of nature is naïve because it ignores the brutality that results from limited resources, the food chain, and the compulsion to survive. In fact, animals in the wild have little freedom, as they are bound to an endless cycle of meeting their basic needs for the purpose of propagating their species. While evolution is often accused of being responsible for this, evolution itself is not a force but a process that encompasses the overall result of biological mechanisms, such as natural selection. In other words, evolution is an effect or result and not a cause. So what then is responsible for limiting the freedom of organisms in nature, and presumably, humans as well?

The answer is genes.

As seen in the study of the cell, genes encoded in DNA are responsible for cellular machinery and processes that keep the cell alive. The influence of genes extends all the way to the organismal level, expressed in the particular traits of an individual. Living things are merely abiding by a molecular set of laws in much the same way that citizens abide by the law of the land. In this sense, genes constitute a set of laws of what is permissible. While organisms in nature must obey the law, humans are increasingly able to attain freedom from their genes through changes in behavior and new medical technologies. But we are only able to have this freedom to a degree, as our genetic government still seems to push for following the natural code of survival and reproduction.

To explore the role of genes as law in anatomy and physiology in this unit, you will investigate the male and female reproductive systems then turn your attention to genetic connections seen through heredity.

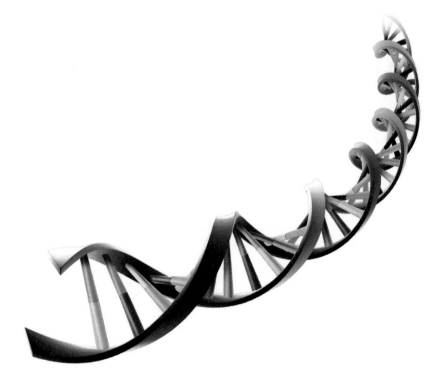

Exercise 18
The Reproductive System

Lesson Overview

Activity #1: Male Reproductive System
Activity #2: Female Reproductive System

Overview

One of the main purposes of a nation's education system is to make children aware of the rules and regulations that govern the country or state they were born into. The process of learning about laws typically starts at an early age and can continue long into adulthood, depending on a person's vocation. Ideally, this education should produce citizens able to participate in their own government. As each generation of students become teachers, voters, lawmakers, and judges, the law is upheld, modified, and passed on.

In a similar way, reproduction is a mechanism that accomplishes related biological goals: the production of offspring and the propagation of genes. While we might not think of reproduction as being a way to participate in the governance of the human genome, that is effectively what we do when we select mates and produce offspring. In essence, the male and female reproductive systems are the anatomical means by which genetic laws are passed on.

Activity #1 — Male Reproductive System

Introduction

The male reproductive system is both a manufacturing facility and a delivery device for the millions of sperm generated each day. In this activity, you will study the structures of the male reproductive system.

Materials

Model of a male reproductive system
Slide of seminiferous tubules and of mouse testes
Posters
Microscope

Procedure

1. Review content in your textbook related to the male reproductive system.
2. The testes are the primary sex organs of the male reproductive system and are housed within the scrotum. Inside the testes, sperm containing 23 chromosomes are produced within the seminiferous tubules in a process known as *spermatogenesis*.

These tubules empty into the rete testis. On the outside of the testis are coiled tubules called the *epididymis*. Examine the prepared microscope slide of the seminiferous tubules in the wall of the testes. Also examine the slide of the rat testes and identify the relevant structures.

3. As the smallest cells of the human body, sperm need a lot of energy to travel long distances and survive for days. Numerous mitochondria fueled by the fructose in semen produce the energy for the flagellating tail. Label the important anatomical features involved in the development and structure of sperm in Figure 18.2.

4. Sperm mature in the epididymis and are stored in the vas deferens up to a month.

The various support fluids called *semen*, which aids in the delivery of sperm, are secreted by the seminal vesicles and prostate. The bulbourethral glands secrete alkaline fluid to neutralize residual urea and lubricate the urethra to minimize the shear forces on sperm during ejaculation, which releases 300-500 million sperm at a time. Once propelled into the vagina through the penis, these millions of sperm are reduced to merely thousands as many succumb to the harsh conditions meant to destroy bacteria. At the same time, the female cervix produces mucus strands for sperm to follow, drawing them upward to promote entry. Identify the anatomical features of the male reproductive system in Figure 18.3.

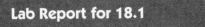

Section A. Male Reproductive System

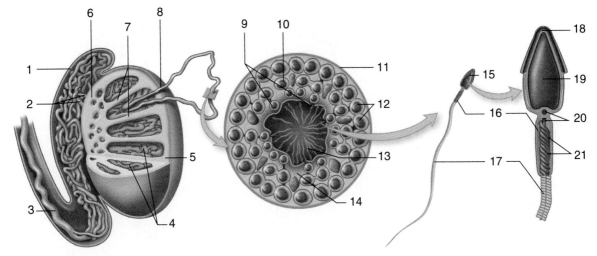

Figure 18.2

Relevant Terms		
_____ Acrosome	_____ Mature sperm cell	_____ Spermatids
_____ Basement membrane	_____ Midpiece	_____ Spermatocyte
_____ Centrioles	_____ Mitochondria	_____ Spermatogonia
_____ Efferent ductules	_____ Nucleus	_____ Sustentacular cell
_____ Epididymis	_____ Rete testis	_____ Tail
_____ Head	_____ Seminiferous tubule	_____ Tunica albuginea
_____ Lobules	_____ Septa	_____ Vas deferens

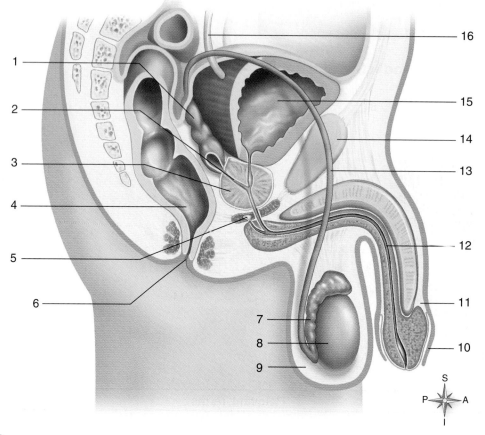

Figure 18.3

Relevant Terms	
_____ Anus	_____ Rectum
_____ Bulbourethral (Cowper) gland	_____ Scrotum
_____ Ejaculatory duct	_____ Seminal vesicle
_____ Epididymis	_____ Testis
_____ Foreskin (prepuce)	_____ Ureter
_____ Penis	_____ Urethra
_____ Prostate gland	_____ Urinary bladder
_____ Pubic symphysis	_____ Vas (ductus) deferens

Section B. Assessments

1. T/F   The primary sex organ of the male reproductive system is the penis.
2. T/F   Seminal fluid is slightly alkaline.
3. The number of sperm cells ejaculated at one time is about:
   a   3 million–5 million.
   b. 30 million–50 million.
   c. 300 million–500 million.
   d. 3 billion–5 billion.
4. The tube that leaves the scrotal sac and enters the abdominal cavity is the:
   a. epididymis.
   b. vas deferens.
   c. seminiferous tubules.
   d. seminal vesicles.

Section C. Critical Thinking Problem

1. What are the advantages and disadvantages of generating new sperm every day?

Activity #2 — Female Reproductive System

Introduction

The female reproductive system is the producer of ova, the female gametes, and serves as a support system for the gestation of zygotes resulting from the fusion of sperm and ova. Hormones trigger the release of ova from the ovaries during the menstrual cycle, approximately 2 weeks after the beginning of menses. In this activity, you will investigate the anatomy of the female reproductive system.

Materials

Model of a female reproductive system
Slide of mammalian ovary
Posters
Microscope

Procedure

1. Review content in your textbook related to the female reproductive system.
2. The primary sex organs of the female reproductive system are the ovaries. These two small organs in the pelvic cavity attach to fallopian tubes. Examine the slide of the ovary. Sketch what you observe in your lab report and label the same structures as seen in Figure 18.4, which shows different stages of follicle development.
3. Ovum production, or oogenesis, occurs in the ovary, culminating in the release of an ovum through a ruptured ovarian follicle; this is ovulation. The ovum then travels through the fallopian tube, or oviduct, to the uterus providing an opportunity for sperm that have traveled through the vagina and cervix — the lower portion of the uterus — to initiate conception. The uterus is also the site where the 40-week gestation period occurs and its lining is sloughed monthly in the process known as *menstruation*. The vagina is a muscular canal that releases menses outside of the body, receives sperm during intercourse, and serves as the canal for delivery during birth. Identify the anatomical features of the female reproductive system in Figure 18.5.
4. Because of their importance in providing nutrients to offspring, the mammary glands are often considered when discussing the reproductive system, though technically they are part of the integumentary system. Mammary glands within the female breast consist of multiple glandular lobes surrounded in adipose tissue that open in the surface of the nipple. During lactation, lobules within the lobes form alveoli, which are sacs that produce milky secretions, and these secretions pass through lactiferous ducts to the nipple. Identify the anatomical features of the mammary glands in Figure 18.6.

Lab Report for 18.2

Section A. Female Reproductive System

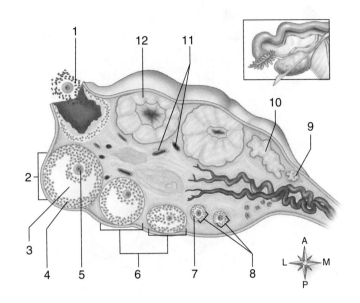

Figure 18.4

Relevant Terms	
_____ Antrum	_____ Granulosa cells
_____ Blood vessels	_____ Mature follicle (Graafian follicle)
_____ Corpus albicans	_____ Oocyte
_____ Corpus luteum	_____ Ovulation
_____ Degenerating corpus luteum	_____ Primary follicles
_____ Granulosa cells	_____ Secondary follicle

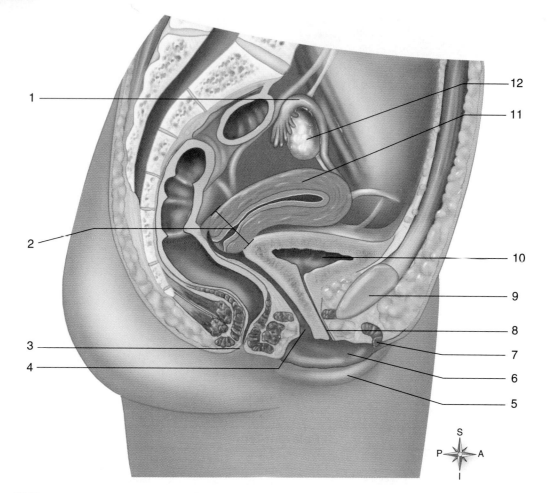

Figure 18.5

Relevant Terms	
_____ Anus	_____ Ovary
_____ Body of uterus	_____ Pubic symphysis
_____ Cervix	_____ Urethra
_____ Clitoris	_____ Urinary bladder
_____ Labium majus	_____ Uterine tube
_____ Labium minus	_____ Vagina

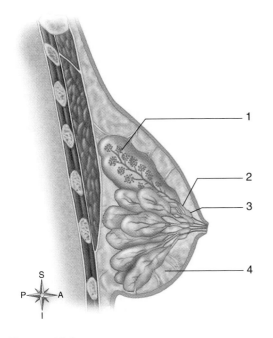

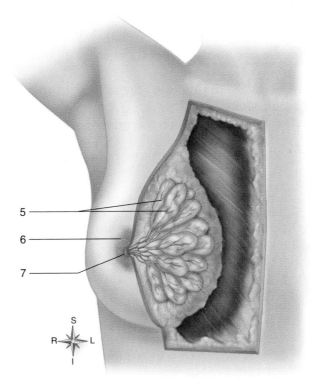

Figure 18.6

Relevant Terms
_____ Adipose tissue
_____ Alveoli
_____ Alveolus
_____ Areola
_____ Lactiferous duct
_____ Lactiferous sinus
_____ Nipple

Section B. Assessments

1. T/F   The uterus is important in the processes of menstruation, pregnancy, and labor.
2. T/F   Milk drains from the alveoli to the lactiferous ducts.
3. The lower portion of the uterus is called the
   a. cervix.
   b. vagina.
   c. ovary.
   d. fallopian tube.
4. Normally, the site of fertilization is the:
   a. ovary.
   b. oviduct.
   c. uterus.
   d. vagina.

Section C. Critical Thinking Problem

1. Female athletes or women involved in routine strenuous exercise may temporarily cease menstruation, a condition known as *amenorrhea*. It turns out that metabolic changes and stress cause hormone release from the hypothalamus to shut down. Interestingly, amenorrhea can also occur in patients with cancer and patients receiving cancer treatment. How is this possible?

Exercise 19
Heredity

Lesson Overview

Activity #1: Genetics and Heredity

Overview

What we are as humans — the structure, order, and organization of our bodies — we owe to our genome. While many of the functions of our genes are slowly being revealed through scientific research, certain physical attributes have always been known to have hereditary links because they could be observed in parents and their offspring. These traits are what we use to describe a person, such as the color of their eyes or what their hair looks like. Other genetic traits are observable but are not commonly used to describe someone, like whether their earlobes are attached or not.

Activity #1 — Genetics and Heredity

Introduction

As you examine your own traits in this lab, reflect on their prevalence in your own family and among the population at large.

Materials

Phenylthiocarbamide (PTC) paper
Astigmatism chart

Procedure

1. Review content in your textbook related to genetics and heredity.

Human Genotypes and Phenotypes

2. The 22 pairs of chromosomes in your cells that are autosomes contain the set of genes inherited from your parents. The same gene at the same location or locus is known as an *allele*. Alleles that are expressed and observable are called *dominant* while those that may be expressed but can be masked are *recessive*. Because chromosomal DNA is packaged in pairs, alleles can exist in one of three forms: *homozygous* dominant (two dominant alleles), homozygous recessive (two recessive alleles) and *heterozygous* (one dominant and one recessive). A set of alleles that an individual has is called a *genotype* while the expression of those alleles into a characteristic is dubbed the *phenotype*. A *trait* is a variant of a phenotype that is distinct, such as blue eyes. When two alleles are neither dominant nor recessive, the relationship is referred to as *codominance*.

   For instance, the widow's peak in the hairline is a dominant trait, so an individual who has a heterozygous genotype, consisting of a dominant *W* allele and a recessive *w* allele, has a *Ww* genotype and thus expresses a widow's peak phenotype.

3. Observe the following phenotypes to determine your genotype and record your results in your lab report.

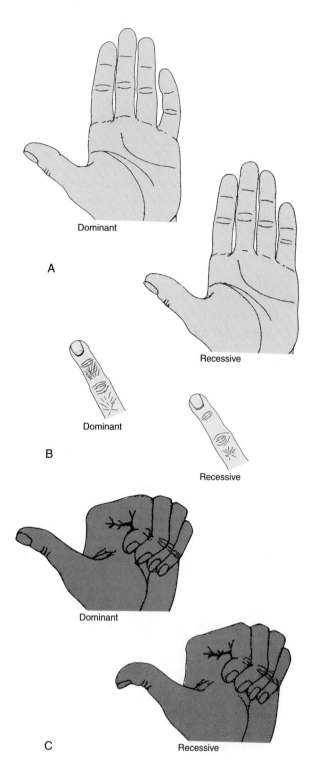

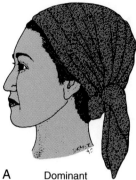

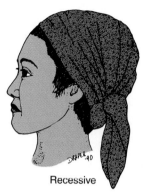

A Dominant   Recessive

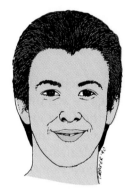

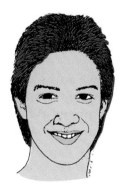

B Dominant   Recessive

C Dominant   Recessive

Sense of Taste

4. *Taster/nontaster (T/t):* PTC paper has a chemical which tastes bitter to about 70% of the population. Place a piece of PTC paper on your tongue and slightly chew it. Record whether you observe a bitter taste. The ability to taste the bitterness is the dominant allele (*T*) and is much stronger for supertasters (*TT*) than for tasters (*Tt*) alone. The recessive phenotype (*tt*) is a nontaster.

Hand Characteristics

5. *Uppermost left/right thumb (L/l):* Clasp your hands together interlocking your fingers and observe which thumb is on top. If the left thumb is the uppermost thumb, you have at least one of the dominant alleles (*L*), but it is not possible to tell if you have both dominant alleles.

6. *Hitchhiker's thumb (H/h):* Make a fist and hold your thumb up. If you can hyperextend the distal joint of your thumb, you have the recessive trait (*hh*).

7. *Angled/straight fifth finger (A/a):* Place your relaxed left hand on the table. If the terminal phalanx of the fifth finger bends toward the fourth finger, you have a dominant allele (*A*).

Hair Characteristics

8. *Widow's peak/straight hairline (W/w):* The presence of a widow's peak in the hairline is a dominant trait (*W*).

9. *Curly/straight hair (C/c):* Curls in untreated hair is a dominant allele (*C*), although in some populations including Caucasians, the heterozygous genotype expresses as a wavy phenotype.

10. *Blaze (B/b):* The presence of a lock of untreated hair with a different color than the rest is a dominant allele (*B*).

Eye Features

11. *Iris color (I/i):* Pigment on the interior and posterior of the iris causes eyes to be green, hazel, or brown. This is the dominant allele (*I*). Blue eye color is due to the recessive trait (*ii*).

12. *Astigmatism/normal vision (S/s):* An abnormal curvature in the lens or cornea of the eye is a dominant allele (*S*). Test for the presence of astigmatism by facing an astigmatism chart similar to Figure 19.2 from a distance of 20 feet. Test each eye by covering one eye and then stare at the center of the chart. If the radiating lines appear curved or there is a difference in the darkness of the lines, astigmatism may be present.

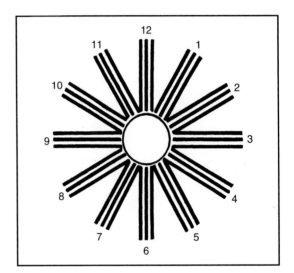

Figure 19.2

Facial Features

13. *Dimples (D/d):* Dimples in one or both cheeks is due to the presence of a dominant allele (*D*).

14. *Freckles (F/f):* Freckles are the result of the dominant allele (*F*).

15. *Attached earlobes (E/e):* If the inferior portion of the earlobe hangs free from the rest of the point of attachment, you have a dominant allele (*E*).

16. *Tongue rolling (R/r):* Extend your tongue. If you can curl your tongue longitudinally into a U shape, you have the dominant allele (*R*) for this trait.

Lab Report for 19.1

Section A. Genetics and Heredity

Record both your phenotype and suspected genotype in the following table:

Trait	Your Phenotype	Possible Genotypes
Sense of taste:		
Hand characteristics:		
Eye characteristics:		
Facial features:		

Section B. Assessments

1. T/F   A genotype is the expression of alleles as a characteristic.
2. T/F   If you can curl your tongue, you have the recessive trait.
3. Which of the following is a homozygous recessive trait?
   a. curls
   b. widow's peak
   c. freckles
   d. hitchhiker's thumb
4. When gametes unite, they form:
   a. an ova.
   b. a zygote.
   c. a spermatozoa.
   d. none of the above.

Section D. Critical Thinking Problem

1. A 2004 study found that almost 500 genes were identical among vertebrates including humans, some of which are so different that their last common ancestor lived 400 million years ago.

   Considering the analogy to law, how would a set of crucial genes compare to certain laws that seem to be present among many different kinds of political systems, such as the laws related to the protection of life and property?